W9-DGJ-389

STUDYING FAMILIES

Applied Social Research Methods Series
Volume 27

APPLIED SOCIAL RESEARCH
METHODS SERIES

Series Editors:
LEONARD BICKMAN, Peabody College, Vanderbilt University, Nashville
DEBRA J. ROG, Vanderbilt University, Washington, DC

STUDYING FAMILIES

Anne P. Copeland
Kathleen M. White

Applied Social Research Methods Series
Volume 27

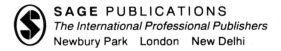

SAGE PUBLICATIONS
The International Professional Publishers
Newbury Park   London   New Delhi

Dedicated to the memory of Aureet Bar-Yam, who epitomized the best in caring relationships and brought many people into her family.

For information address:

SAGE Publications, Inc.
2455 Teller Road
Newbury Park, California 91320

SAGE Publications Ltd.
6 Bonhill Street
London EC2A 4PU
United Kingdom

SAGE Publications India Pvt. Ltd.
M-32 Market
Greater Kailash I
New Delhi 110 048 India

Printed in the United States of America

Library of Congress Cataloging-in-Publication Data

Copeland, Anne P., 1951-
    Studying families / Anne P. Copeland and Kathleen M. White.
        p.   cm. — (Applied social research methods series: v. 27)
    Includes bibliographical references and index.
    ISBN 0-8039-3247-2 (c). — ISBN 0-8039-3248-0 (p)
    1. Family—Research. 2. Family—Research—United States.
  I. White, Kathleen M., 1940-   . II. Title. III. Series.
  HQ503.C67   1991
  306.85′072—dc20
                                  90-11125
                                     CIP

92 93 94 15 14 13 12 11 10 9 8 7 6 5 4 3

Sage Production Editor: Michelle R. Starika

Contents

Foreword

This useful, concise book is about something old and something very new. The old is represented by the family, and the acknowledgment that the family is a crucible in which individual development, group behavior, and society intersect. What is new, however, is that the family is no longer the focus of one discipline within the social sciences. During the past decade or two, there has been an explosion of interest in the family from many disciplines, and one of the exciting developments in this field is the stimulation of interest in the family through interdisciplinary research.

Although it is easy to extol the virtues of interdisciplinary research, the realities of doing such work are very difficult. Oftentimes, researchers find themselves called upon to be "bilingual" or "multilingual" in being able to speak the languages and use the techniques of different disciplines in their own work. The study of the family has focused a need for distinctive research methods, since a family is neither simply a collection of individuals nor just another social group. Family researchers have identified specific issues dealing with theory and methodology that are unique to this particular enterprise.

This volume by Copeland and White makes a major contribution to the family scholars of the present and future. The goal of *Studying Families* is to provide a concise treatment of the special issues and problems relating to research on families. It should be a welcome resource to students of the family from different disciplinary persuasions.

Studying Families begins by acknowledging that special problems are encountered when one wishes to treat the family as the level of analysis. It immediately moves the reader away from an oversimplified assumption that methods developed for studying individuals are directly applicable to studying the family. The book includes useful overviews of different types of research techniques, including both self-report and observational methods. In addition, it focuses on the issues involved in assessing individuals, relationships, or families, and what may be learned from making these assessments on the basis of asking individuals or families. Two of the chapters are particularly unique. One discusses the advantage for family scholars of using existing data sources for answering research questions. As the cost of conducting research escalates and the availability of resources declines, it simply makes good sense to take the best advantage of data already collected in the field. Copeland and White provide some stimulating suggestions on how to do this, although they are also realistic in evaluating the pitfalls involved in the use of secondary data. Chapter 6 addresses some of the thorny issues involved in applying traditional statistical techniques to the study of families. In a nontechnical way, the authors outline the considerations that must be taken into account when aggregating data at the family level and performing the desired analyses.

Throughout the book, the authors convey the message that the study of the family is an exciting and vibrant area of investigation but that, at the same time, it presents unique and demanding challenges to the researcher. *Studying Families* should go a long way toward helping family scholars from different disciplinary backgrounds identify key issues with which they must grapple. In many ways, it will contribute positively to family researchers' finding common ground for their scientific work.

Harold D. Grotevant, Ph.D.
Professor and Head
Department of Family Social Science
University of Minnesota

Acknowledgments

This book was written in the context of the family research training program in the Psychology Department of Boston University, where graduate students and faculty members from our programs in clinical, personality, developmental, and social psychology join in considering methodological, theoretical, and personal aspects of doing family research. We are indebted to this group for many of the ideas in this book and for first establishing the opportunity to collaborate with each other.

In addition, we would like to thank Abigail Stewart, Daniel Ozer, and an anonymous reviewer for their helpful comments on the manuscript. We share any credit with them, and of course accept responsibility ourselves.

1

Introduction

David and Nancy's family had always been close. They planned fun activities for their whole family on weekends, and their four children, closely spaced in age, seemed to thrive when they were young. The community admired them, and many envied them. As each child reached adolescence, however, various troubles arose. Julie, the oldest, dropped out of high school for a year. Ben, next in line, was in a car crash involving drunk driving. Kristen seemed to shine in high school and college, though her participation in some activities was limited because of undiagnosed recurrent headaches. As the older children moved out of the home, Natalie, the youngest, became increasingly thin, and was finally diagnosed as anorexic. In order to help her eat right and get back on her feet, her parents set up a small apartment for her on their third floor. When the Jacksons appeared at the University Family Research Laboratory to participate in a study on Families with Young Adult Children, Natalie, age 27, was working for her father and living in the third-floor apartment. Julie lived far from home and rarely communicated with the family. Ben lived nearby with his wife, who did not get along with her in-laws. And Kristen had what seemed to be an ideal husband, an ideal baby, and an ideal job. Nancy, their mother, had taken a job that required her to travel most of the week, and David and Natalie spent most of their time together.

How should the researchers describe this family? The traditional psychological method would be to assess each member's personality or behavior or living situation, or perhaps to study one randomly chosen child and his/her interactions with the parents or siblings. But in this case, everyone seems so different. What could be done with the diversity? Would it make sense to ask each of the children about their view of the family, add up the scores, and divide by four? Would it be valid to conclude something about the family by simply describing the relationship between one randomly chosen parent and one randomly chosen child? Specifically, what if this turned out to be David and Natalie's relationship? Nancy and Julie's? Is there really some common important trait that the family members do, in fact, continue to share? Where should the researchers look if they want to account for the difference in outcomes of the four children? Is Julie's experience influenced by her

1

being the oldest of these particular four children? Did David and Nancy's marital relationship change as the children each grew up, so that each child reached young adulthood with parents in a different state of marital satisfaction? Is Nancy's current distance from the family a cause or an effect of her husband and youngest daughter's closeness? Or both?

These are the kinds of questions family researchers are trying to tackle. Certainly, family researchers use many of the traditional techniques used in psychology; the foundations of observational coding, test construction and psychometrics, and statistics, for example, form an integral part of the family researcher's tools. Indeed, many important questions about families can be addressed using existing, traditional methods. But family research is not simply a matter of using traditional methods that were developed to study individuals to study members of a family. Rather, it also marks a major paradigm shift: a conceptual, methodological, and statistical departure from traditional methods by refocusing on different units of analysis; on nonlinear, multifactorial, and indirect models of causality; and/or on the process of change.

For the family researcher, the diversity of David and Nancy's children might become the central focus of interest, rather than being seen as a point to be mentioned as an anecdote in a discussion section of an article. Or, the focus might be on describing or predicting the development of this family from the early idyllic days of young childhood through the rocky adolescent period to the current stage of young adulthood, or on the interplay between the parents' relationship with each other and with each child, or on the broader context of community forces and ethnic background, or the role of extended family in affecting the development of family members. Thus, unlike the traditional psychological focus on individuals, the focus of family research is on some larger unit. One might ask, then, exactly what "counts" as a family, and how families are different from other small groups that psychologists have studied.

WHAT IS A FAMILY?

At first glance, this may seem to be an easy question. Easy answer: the mother, the father, and the children. But, of course, families come in many different forms these days, and the so-called "traditional" family that consists of two parents married to each other and their biological children is becoming proportionally less and less common. Enormous social change in the past several decades has raised new questions about what constitutes a "family" and has challenged previous conclusions based on the traditional definitions. Family constellations that were once rare (blended families, homosexual parenting, never-married mothers) are now more common, and they need to be better understood. Demographic changes, including a broadening of the age range (in both directions) during which women marry or have children, a decrease in numbers of full-time homemakers, and an increase in single-parent families, make much of psychological research on children, marriage, and families outdated or at least limited in generalizability. Thus even the very first practical question that faces a researcher—who shall be included in the study—has become a complex issue. Consider the following questions:

1. Should non-nuclear family members sharing the home be included? For example, what if a grandmother lives in the home? What if she does most of the child rearing? What about an uncle? A boarder? A boarder who has lived there for 10 years? A boarder who has lived there for 2 weeks?
2. What about children who have left home, say, to go to college? To get married? Is it different if they live in town and drop in every day or live across the country and visit one weekend a year?
3. Do the child-rearing adults in the family have to be married to each other to be included in the definition of a family? At what point does a mother's boyfriend become a father substitute? What about homosexual partners?
4. In single-parent families, does the "family" include the noncustodial parent? What if there is joint custody? If both parents have remarried, is the child considered to have two families?
5. In step- and reconstituted families, how soon after marriage is the new family considered the meaningful family for the members? Immediately? After a month? A year?
6. Does more than one generation have to be represented to count as a family? What about married couples? Couples without children?
7. Under what conditions, if any, should a family with adopted or foster children be considered separately from a family with biological children?

These are just some of the questions that may arise in trying to define a sample or a framework for understanding family process. With recent social change has come a new empowerment of groups of people, such as women, homosexuals, and minorities, who are questioning some of the assumptions and theoretical frameworks of much of the existing psychological literature, and who are in a position to define *family* in new ways, conduct new research studies, ask new questions, and ask old questions in a different way. We do not propose to set limits of inclusion or exclusion about what counts as a family for family research. Each investigator's answer should be based on a sound, conceptual reason, for it will have methodological, statistical, and interpretive consequences.

For example, if one is interested in the role that family expectations, myths, and history have on a child, one might include information from or about parents or grandparents who have died or even who have never been known to the child, and exclude nonrelated people living in the home. If instead, one is interested in day-to-day conflict styles, one might make the opposite choice about inclusion. It is important to be clear about the rationale for the choices one makes in any particular study, but faulty to think that any one definition will be appropriate across the field of family research.

HOW FAMILY RESEARCH DIFFERS FROM RESEARCH WITH OTHER SMALL GROUPS

Despite the undesirability of hard-and-fast rules about "what is a family," however, there are certain characteristics of families that should be considered when designing family research. Families are not just some random collection of people, gathered together for a moment's participation in a research study. Thus, while we can stand on the shoulders of others who have studied groups of people, several considerations should be taken into account.

For example, social psychology, in its study of small group process, has added considerably to the study of family interaction. The issues of dominance, power, acceptance of and resistance to change, and leadership, for example, have all been studied by social psychologists and have informed the field of family research in terms of both conceptual models and observational tools. However, social psychologists usually focus on nonfamily groups, like groups at work, dormitory groups, or groups formed temporarily, purely for the purpose of the research study. Families are different from these groups in fundamental ways, ways that limit the utility of the methods and concepts used by social psychologists.

First, families have a shared history. The history stretches back for generations and involves ethnic or religious values. The participants in a family research study bring to every interaction expectations about each other based on extended prior experience and family myth. Of course, these expectations are often unstated, maybe even denied, but are inalterably present nevertheless. Thus turn-taking in conversation might be dictated by the rule, accepted by all in the family but spoken by none, "Let mother answer the questions. She's the reflective one, not father. He's just like all the men in the family." These kinds of entrenched expectations do not exist to the same extent in ad hoc research groups and other naturally formed groups. When family interaction process is the focus of the research, however, it should not be ignored by the researcher any more than it should or could be by the family members.

Families also have a shared future. What happens in the laboratory may not be chalked up to "an interesting experience" and forgotten the next day, and everyone in the family knows it. Especially in studies in which families are asked to discuss important, real issues together, the promises of anonymity and confidentiality about what they say, usually afforded to research subjects, are limited because the other family members are sitting there and listening. This alters the kinds of questions a researcher asks and the kinds of interpretations that can be made of the resulting data. There is also a special responsibility of the researcher to attend to the effect of the study on the family.

Third, some members of families have a shared biology. The degree to which temperament, personality, talent, or behavior are inherited is unclear, but the potential for a biological bias toward intermember similarity is certainly greater in families than in other kinds of groups.

There is also a built-in power hierarchy in families that is less obvious or nonexistent in other groups. This hierarchy is partially determined by the existence of two or more generations, partially by culture-wide expectations (e.g., for different sexes), partially by age differences even within a generation, and partially by idiosyncratic family history. The roles of parents and children define their behavior (even when roles appear to be reversed), and make observational code systems that assume equality moot.

CONCLUSION AND OUTLINE

We have tried to introduce the reader to the kinds of questions family researchers ask and to discuss some of the problems that ensue from the answers to these questions. The purpose of the rest of this book is to detail the ways in which questions being asked about families are different from questions about individuals, and to describe the traditional, the new, and the to-be-developed tools needed to address these questions. While many of our examples are psychological in nature, reflecting our own backgrounds, the issues raised in this book are relevant for family researchers from many perspectives. Throughout, we try to focus on the special problems of family researchers, referring the reader to other sources for discussion of issues that family researchers share with other disciplines. In Chapter 2, we discuss some general aspects of family research design and measurement choice. Chapters 3 and 4 focus on self-report and observational approaches to collecting family data, while in Chapter 5 we discuss ways to study families without collecting new data. Chapter 6 reviews some of the data analysis issues that arise in family research. And in Chapter 7 we try to frame the challenges of the field as it stands now and prepare a new generation of family researchers to make new contributions.

EXERCISES

1. Develop a description of another family, like that of David and Nancy. Write at least five research questions that might be asked about them from an individual perspective, and then write at least five research questions about them from a family perspective. What statistical and methodological problems would you face in posing your family questions? Do you have solutions for these problems?
2. Think of a family research topic, and write the inclusion and exclusion criteria for participants in this study. Refer to the list in the "What Is a Family" section of this chapter. Think about who would be important to include in the study and why.

RECOMMENDED READING

Bell, R. Q. (1965). A reinterpretation of the direction of effects in studies of socialization. *Psychological Review, 75,* 81-95.

Kaye, K. (1985). Toward a developmental psychology of the family. In L. L'Abate (Ed.), *The handbook of family psychology and therapy* (Vol. 1, pp. 38-72). Homewood, IL: Dorsey.

Miller, D. R., & Sobelman, G. (1985). Models of the family: A critical review of alternatives. In L. L'Abate (Ed.), *The handbook of family psychology and therapy* (Vol. 1, pp. 3-37). Homewood, IL: Dorsey.

2

Designing Family Research

Although many aspects of family research design and execution parallel those of more traditional approaches, some special problems exist in the study of families, for several reasons. First, since the field is so new, one must begin by asking fundamental questions about theory and model validation. What are the dimensions on which families differ from each other, and how do we decide which of these dimensions are critical to an understanding of development and mental health? Where do researchers derive their ideas for family studies? Are quantitative, traditional methods of social science inquiry the only or the best methods for addressing the complexity of families?

Second, certain methodological problems arise when one tries to draw conclusions about families since they are made up of multiple individuals who change over time. Can we use individuals' reports to tell us anything about whole families? What do we do if our various informants disagree with each other? What does it mean if individuals' reports about their families change from day to day? What kinds of research designs can capture between-family differences and within-family changes in family interaction? These issues are discussed briefly in this chapter (readers will also be interested in an extended discussion of them in Christensen & Arrington [1987]).

FUNDAMENTAL ISSUES IN
MODEL DEVELOPMENT AND
METHODS OF INQUIRY

What sources do investigators use for framing meaningful research questions about families? As in all areas of research, a first step is to consider the *theoretical and empirical work* of other researchers. Conceptual models built on a set of general principles about the family can suggest new ways of understanding a problem. Moreover, theoretically driven research is likely to help prevent the development of a literature full of ad hoc and idiosyncratic explanations of family issues (see

Grotevant, 1989, for a discussion of the need for and state of theory-driven research).

A large number of different proposals have been made to describe normal and pathogenic family process. These differ widely in the assumptions they make about what is "healthy," the dimensions they consider to be of primary importance, and the process through which they presume families function. The role of families in the development of psychopathology, for example, has been approached from a variety of perspectives, including behavioral genetics (Pogue-Geile & Rose, 1987), social learning (Robinson & Jacobson, 1987), developmental (B. Martin, 1987), and systemic (Steinglass, 1987) ones.

General Systems Theory (von Bertalanffy, 1968), the basis of most family therapy and many family process theories, specifies that families, like many groups (e.g., basketball teams, work groups, countries), share a number of characteristics with some other biological systems: the system (family) has its own characteristics that are not simply the sum of the individual members' traits, all parts (people) are interdependent on each other even though the parts (people) have different roles or places in a hierarchy, feedback loops function to keep the system in a relatively stable state, and exchange of information and adaptation occur both within the system (family) and between the system and broader environment (community).

This systemic approach has led to a method of treating psychological problems and of posing research questions that is fundamentally different from the traditional, individually based one. The target individual's role in the family is emphasized rather than individual psychopathology, and subtle and pervasive reciprocity or circularity of causation is assumed to occur. For example, a young man's continued unemployment and refusal to leave home might be treated not in terms of some individual disorder, but rather in terms of its function for the family—if he left home and were successful, would the parents' now-childless marriage survive? General systems theory has had a great influence on the field of family research, marking as it does a major shift in assumptions about causality and reciprocity, but it is only one of many important theories. The interested reader is referred to Burr, Hill, Nye, and Reiss (1979a, 1979b), Thomas and Wilcox (1987), or Jacob (1987) for thorough lists and descriptions of comprehensive family models.

Against the backdrop of a major theoretical perspective, most researchers work within some narrower framework that focuses on a specific aspect of family process (Grotevant, 1989). For example, Olson and his colleagues (Olson, Sprenkle, & Russell, 1979) have described a Circumplex Model that focuses attention on family members' reports of *cohesion* (the closeness or emotional bonding that family members have toward one another) and *adaptability* (the family's ability to change the power structure, role relationships, and relationship rules in response to situational and developmental stress). Mid-range levels of cohesion and adaptability are thought to be optimal, while extreme levels of either dimension are thought to be maladaptive.

Reiss (1981), in describing a Paradigm Model, focuses on *configuration* (family members' view of the social environment as ordered and understandable or as disordered and baffling, and whether they view themselves as capable of mastering the environment or as helpless), *coordination* (family members' view of themselves as a relatively loosely connected group of autonomous individuals or as a unitary, bounded group), and *closure* (family members' view of themselves as developing and changing with experience or as continuous with its past traditions, and whether the environment is viewed as novel and intriguing or continually familiar). Families are described in terms of how they experience the extrafamilial environment (e.g., how they use cues from the external and intrafamily environment, how highly they value family cohesiveness, how much they share perceptions and hypotheses about problem solving) as reflected in their behavior during a problem-solving task.

Beavers (1976) suggests that families fall on an "infinite continuum" of competence, a function of family structure, family mythology, goal-directed negotiation, autonomy, and affective expression. On one side of the continuum are families that are leaderless and chaotic, and who have diffuse interpersonal boundaries. On the other side are well-structured families made up of autonomous individuals who share intimacy and closeness easily yet have respect for each member's separateness.

In describing the McMaster Model of Family Functioning, Epstein, Bishop, and Levine (1978) proposed that family behavior can be described along the dimensions of problem solving (how instrumental and affective problems are dealt with), communication (whether information is exchanged in clear and direct ways), roles (repetitive patterns of behavior by which individuals fulfill their functions), affective responsiveness (families' ability to respond to a range of stimuli with appropriate quality and quantity of feelings), affective involvement (interest shown in and value given to activities and interests of family members), and behavior control (how families deal with physically dangerous situations, psychobiological needs, and socializing behavior). Object relations theory and the close-relationships framework mark two other psychological perspectives on family process (Grotevant, 1989). *Personal experience* is another tempting source of research ideas in the study of families. Everybody has a family, and everybody has notions about how families work. Every family deals with such issues as closeness versus distance, independence versus dependence, and differences of opinion, power, and authority, so we all have developed some implicit or explicit hypotheses about family functioning. Further, many of us have firsthand knowledge of how some particular experience can affect families, experiences such as having a member with AIDS, adoption, birth of a retarded child, unemployment, or being an immigrant. These experiences often enable us to propose meaningful and useful research questions. As families continue to undergo changes in structure and function and to encounter new problems that have not been studied before, fresh perspectives on families will be particularly important.

While it is true that firsthand knowledge can lead to intuition and insight about family process, there are also disadvantages to relying exclusively on personal experience, especially the personal experience of just one person, for hypothesis generation and data collection plans. Personal experience can limit the types of questions asked and may lead to distortions in interpretation. For example, suppose an investigator grew up in a family in which the mother was the "emotional" one and the father the "clear-headed and rational" one, and the investigator grew to feel that this was an inhibiting pattern for optimal child development. She might set out to test ("prove") this hypothesis, focusing on these two patterns to the exclusion of other potentially important dimensions of parenting style. Conversely, she might accept this parental pattern, even unwittingly, as the "norm." In designing a study about parental interaction with children, she might therefore ask questions, pose tasks, and have coding biases consistent with these stereotypes. In her study a father who hugged his child might be coded as "unusually emotional," or a planful, organized mother as "overfunctioning and cold."

While social scientists strive to be "value free" and to eschew preconceptions, in fact this is very difficult to do. The recent debate in psychology about whether women's experience is represented adequately in theories and research advanced by, and with, men highlights this dilemma. It is a particularly difficult issue in family research because of the salience of our own family histories. It is perhaps easier for researchers of "reaction time" or "selective attention" to keep personal biases out of the laboratory than it is for investigators of family process. Thus one admonition for family researchers is to be aware continually of their values and assumptions, and to plan research in consultation with others from differing backgrounds.

A more radical response to the issue of values in science is to adopt a *qualitative* rather than or in addition to the traditional *quantitative* approach to theory development, methodology, and analysis. While qualitative research is still relatively new in the field of family research, it is consistent with a systemic perspective and we expect to see more and more of it in the near future (see Fetterman, 1989; also Sprey, 1988, for a discussion of the role of qualitative methods in theories about families; Reinharz, 1984, for a description of qualitative research; and Jayaratne & Stewart, in press, for a discussion of combining qualitative and quantitative approaches).

Specifically, qualitative researchers emphasize involvement, mutuality, and rapport between participants and themselves (as opposed to establishing a more distant, one-sided relationship as is the case in traditional research) in the belief that they get more realistic, valid, and important information in doing so. Qualitative research often involves small samples of participants who are interviewed and observed, or, more accurately, are "visited" in the natural environment (e.g., their own homes) on many occasions. Data usually consist of open-ended remarks made in the context of interview conversations between participants and researchers. Participants also may be asked their views on the way the topic is being studied, and the qualitative researcher may alter her method in response to input from participants. Rather than assess families at several different discrete points in time in a traditional longitudinal design, qualitative researchers are more likely to be involved intensely with particpants throughout a time period, watching change unfold before them. These data are later used to describe patterns, emergent concepts, and themes, as opposed to being coded into predetermined categories. Thus data collection is, by design, part of the process of theory-building, rather than being a method of theory-testing. It is also common for qualitative researchers to consider the participants (and the population from which they were drawn) a legitimate and important audience for their writing, as opposed to writing exclusively for the scientific community (Reinharz, 1984).

An excellent example of qualitative research is Hochschild's (1989) interview study of 10 couples with children in which both husbands and wives were employed outside the home. The focus was on the simple question of who did the housework and child care in the family. Using the information she obtained through intensive and personal interviews, Hochschild was able to interpret themes in the couples' stories within a broad framework that included participants' gender ideologies, family histories, and the competing demands of current social standards. In short, qualitative research represents a challenge to many of the assumptions of quantitative research approaches. While the remainder of this book focuses primarily on more traditional quantitative methods, reflecting the predominant approach to date in the field of family research, we anticipate discovering new kinds of knowledge about families, obtained in new ways through qualitative methods, in the near future.

Informed by theory, then, and enlightened by and appropriately wary of one's own biases, the next step in getting started is to *learn what other investigators have found* about a particular topic and how they have studied it. Table 2.1 provides a list of the major family journals. The *Family Studies Abstracts* (published by Sage) can be particularly useful in providing references on family topics. Each issue is organized into major topic areas (e.g., marriage, family and society, sexual attitudes and behavior, sex roles, issues concerning reproduction, marriage and mate selection, the family life cycle, and family relations and communication). Each issue also has both an author index and a subject index that provide the numbers of the abstracts in that issue featuring that author or topic.

Another useful source for finding articles about issues of interest is the Sage publication, *Inventory of Marriage and Family Literature.* Published annually since 1980 and a few times before that date, that publication lists current references relevant to various family issues. In the 1988 volume, for example, under the subject heading "Alternate Family Forms," complete bibliographic references are listed for such articles as "Changes in Family Functioning Amongst Nonconventional Families," "Adoption as a Means of Family Formation," and "On Conflict in Nontraditional Families—A Clinical Perspective."

A number of useful volumes have been published recently that compile various methods for measuring family constructs (e.g., Grotevant & Carlson, 1988; Touliatos, Perlmutter, & Straus, 1989). Also, we have found the following to be of particular use in summarizing the state of the art in family research, from both methodological and theoretical points of view: Jacob (1987), L'Abate (1985), and Grotevant & Carlson (1988).

Table 2.1

Journals Primarily Focused on Family Issues

Title	Professional Association/Publisher
Journal of Family Psychology	American Psychological Association
Journal of Marriage and the Family	National Council on Family Relations
Family Process	Family Process, Inc.
Journal of Family Issues	Sage: National Council on Family Relations
Family Relations	National Council on Family Relations
Journal of Family History	National Council on Family Relations
Family Studies Abstracts	Sage Publications

MODEL VALIDATION
THROUGH MULTIPLE MEASUREMENT

The initial task in a new field like family psychology is establishing exactly which constructs one thinks are important to study. Once one's research question is established and justified, the next step is to plan a study that will examine that question. Of course, the procedures for conducting research on families are in many ways the same as those for conducting research on individuals. One devises a way to measure the construct(s) of interest, assesses the reliability and validity of the measures, chooses an appropriate sample, and then tests the hypotheses to see if the model holds up under relevant conditions. However, partly because family research is a new field and partly because of some of its inherent characteristics, some of these issues are problematic in different ways for family researchers, as discussed below.

Once one has decided what to study, one needs to decide how to measure it. Unfortunately, there are few examples in family research of constructs that are clearly captured by well-established and widely accepted measures (see Chapters 3 and 4 for some exceptions). This may be because many of the constructs of interest in the study of the family are of an internal, symbolic, and/or subtle behavioral nature, aspects of human psychology that have traditionally been difficult to capture quantitatively. The approach many investigators have used to address these problems is to use more than one measure of a given construct, assuming more measures will assess the construct more reliably and fully than a simple measure. Some researchers ask more than one person to complete the same measure in an attempt to get a more complete description of the phenomenon. Others try to assess different but related constructs to try to capture the breadth of the issue.

Still others have used divergent approaches to the measurement of the same construct to try to assess robustness. As discussed in the following sections, however, each of these approaches has met with difficulty.

Having Two Judges Complete the Same Measure

Traditionally, when two judges (e.g., two parents, two teachers, two clinicians) have been used in research studies, the purpose has been to assess the psychometric properties of the measures used. Lack of comparability has been interpreted as a fault in the measure—that is, poor interrater reliability. The rationale is that if a subject characteristic is measurable and the measure is a good one, all users of the measure ought to come up with the same score for a given subject. However, a different interpretation of lack of interrater comparability is possible. Two family members may give different assessments of a particular family characteristic not because the measurement device is a poor one, but because their perspectives on the characteristic are different. For example, husbands and wives may have different feelings about the quality of their marriage (see Bernard, 1982, for a description of "his" and "her" marriages), adolescents and younger children may differ in their evaluations of family cohesion, and parents' ratings of a child's behavior problems may differ. In each of these cases, it may be that each rater is accurately describing his or her own perspective on the target characteristic. The standard of comparison might differ between raters (as it might if husbands and wives have different "ideal" marriages in mind when they describe their own). Different developmental issues and abilities might affect how one rates one's family (as it would if adolescents and younger children had different bonds to their family and different degrees of information about what other families are like). Or, the information upon which respondents base their rating might differ (as it would if a mother spends most of her time with a child in daily chores and the father spends most of his time with a child in play).

Achenbach, McConaughy, and Howell (1987) provide a useful discussion of this issue of interrater disagreement. In a meta-analysis of 119 studies in which ratings of behavioral or emotional problems of children by at least two informants were compared, they found that pairs of informants with similar roles with respect to the child (e.g., two parents, two teachers) showed higher agreement (mean $r = .60$) than did pairs of different types of informants (mean $r = .28$) or children themselves with other informants (mean $r = .22$). These results were based on measures with relatively high test-retest reliability and interob-server reliability between simultaneous observations by trained ob-servers (rs in the .80s and .90s). Consistency across informants was generally higher for 6- to 11-year-olds than for adolescents and for ratings of problems of undercontrol (e.g., hyperactivity) compared with overcontrol (e.g., depression, anxiety). The authors concluded that it is desirable to obtain data from more than one informant, while noting that data from one informant is a reasonable estimate of what another informant of the same type might give. Further, it is clear that different informants, especially the children themselves, provide different and distinct types of information. Others have suggested that parents may be less willing to give a negative view of their families to outsiders than are children (Reiss, 1981), and that agreement between family members may differ depending on how "healthy" the family is (Beavers, 1977; Hampson, Beavers, & Hulgus, 1989).

Thus the approach of strengthening one's information about a family by asking two or more members to report becomes a complex issue. Disagreement may not be measurement error, but valuable information to be preserved. What to do statistically with several reports on a given family is discussed in Chapter 6.

Measuring Different but Related Constructs

Because many of the constructs of interest to family researchers are new and because the number of theories used to guide research is large, the field has quickly amassed a large amount of data, in which questions are asked in different ways, and different measures based on different theoretical assumptions are used, yielding different interpretations (see Grotevant & Carlson, 1988, for a useful description and review of many of these measures). Within this amalgam of research is the troubling and pervasive finding of lack of comparability across measures of supposedly similar constructs.

For example, some investigators have compared measures of differ-ent but presumably related family constructs, derived from different theories. The assumption is that two models may target similar family dimensions, even if they call them different names. For example, Reiss and his colleagues compared ratings of families on his card-sorting procedure with self-report ratings on Moos and Moos' Family Environ-ment Scale (Oliveri & Reiss, 1984) and, in a separate study, on the Family Adaptability and Cohesion Evaluation Scales (Sigafoos, Reiss, Rich, & Douglas, 1985). Although the constructs measured with these various tools were admittedly different, the authors argued that because they were conceptually similar and had predicted clinical behavior similarly, they ought to be related when measured in the same families. These predictions were not upheld, however.

Using Divergent Approaches to Measure the Same Construct

Other family researchers have attacked the issue of measurement from many sides at once, standing on the shoulders of both behavioral observers and psychometricians from several disciplines to try to understand family process. (A more complete treatment of the strengths and limits of self-report and observational measures is found in Chapter 3 and 4, respectively.) The question here is the extent to which self-report and observational approaches yield similar conclusions about families.

Working within a single model (the Beavers Systems model), Hampson et al. (1989) rated 110 two-parent families on observational measures of *competence* (i.e., power relationships, parental coalitions, closeness, mythology, negotiation style, clarity of expression, responsibility, permeability, demonstrated range of affect, mood and tone, presence of unresolvable conflict, empathy, and global health) and *style* (i.e., handling of dependency needs, style of adult conflict, proximity, social presentation, verbal expression of closeness, aggressiveness, expression of feelings, and global centripetal/centrifugal style). They also had family members complete self-report measures of health, conflict, cohesion, leadership, and emotional expression, which are presumed to be the major elements of competence and style. Overall, correlations between self-reports and observers' ratings of competence and style were significant for fathers, mothers, and adolescents (ranging from .35 to .79). Thus working within the same conceptual model, these authors reported a significant degree of congruence across measurement methods.

The assumption of this approach is that the constructs being measured ought to be captured both phenomenologically and behaviorally. Unless the model presumes that the construct is either fully accessible to the family members themselves (and therefore able to be reported by them) or can be tapped through indirect self-report (such that the investigator gives meaning to the person's responses that he or she may not have intended) and that the construct can be expected to be elicited in the observation setting, this assumption is a tenuous one. The issue of agreement across different measurement strategies has concerned family researchers for a number of years and has yielded a range of perspectives on the problem.

Olson (1977) noted that self-report and observational methods differ in whether they reveal an "insider's" (self-report) or "outsider's" (observer's) perspective on the family. Sigafoos et al. (1985) make the interesting suggestion that if one considers the social context in which research data are collected—that is, the relationship between the researcher and the subject(s)—self-report measures about families and observational measures differ radically. When individuals are asked to report their views of their family (privately, to the outsider researcher), they are necessarily responding to their perception of what the researcher wants to know about or to hear. In addition, the implicit message when a researcher asks an individual for his or her view of the family (as in a self-report) is that the two of them stand apart from the rest of the family in capturing its real essence. In contrast, observations of entire families put all family members together, with the researcher clearly the outsider. Especially when the task given to the family is ambiguous in meaning, family members are less tempted and less able to try to respond to outsiders' expectations, and instead they have no choice but to apply their own "construction of reality" on the situation. (Olson and Sigafoos and Reiss have an interesting exchange of papers in the June 1985 issue of *Family Process* on these interpretations of the meaning of self-report and observations in family research.)

In discussing the meaning of the lack of convergence of measurement across different methods in personality research, Ozer (1989) suggests that, in some cases, the use of different methods (e.g., self-report and observational ones) connotes inherently different theoretical assumptions about the construct at hand, and that one would not necessarily expect convergence of results across measures. Further, he suggests that measurement scores must be construed as a reflection of both the trait and the method used to measure it (as opposed to the more traditional interpretation of a score as a reflection of the trait, distorted to some degree by the method).

Further, Huston and Robins (1982) propose a distinction between *subjective conditions* (relatively stable attitudes, attributes, and beliefs that an individual has either about another member of the family or about their relationship) and *relationship properties* (recurrent patterns of interpersonal or subjective events). They suggest that self-report is the most appropriate way to assess subjective conditions and that behavioral observations are the method of choice when one is interested in relationship properties; lack of agreement between the two methods could be a reflection of a faulty match between method and construct. Another important dimension in understanding this problem is whether family members and observers share a view on the meaning of the constructs. For example, Hampson et al. (1989) found that self-reports of family "cohesion" on the FACES II measure (supposedly a measure that could pick up the clinically distinct aspects of enmeshment, or overinvolvement, and disengagement, or underinvolvement) were more highly correlated with family idealization and "prizing" one's family than with clinical ratings of enmeshment.

To the extent that many of the concepts of interest to family researchers involve both the individuals' own perceptions and their behavior, this issue of the relationship between self-report and behavioral observation will continue to be an important one in this field. More generally, the problem of how to make sense of information obtained from various sources, measured with different approaches, and based on different assumptions is a continuing one in family research (see Chamberlain & Bank, 1989, for a discussion of this issue).

RELIABILITY AND VALIDITY

Reliability

Like all other social researchers, family researchers must be concerned with the reliability (consistency, as between two scorers, two forms of the measure, or two testings) of the measures in their studies. The reader is referred to Anastasi (1988) for a description of reliability and validity issues in psychological research. However, two points are worthy of special attention by family researchers. First, as discussed earlier in this chapter, interrater disagreement should not necessarily be considered a reflection of poor measurement reliability. Second, a parallel concern exists in assessing test-retest reliability. If a measure taps a stable trait, if the measure is reliable, and (with children) if the second assessment is not too far removed from the first, then a person should score about the same on the measure on two different occasions. However, many family theorists suggest that very rigid patterns of interaction in a family (e.g., the father always leads any discussion and the mother always acquiesces) are indicators of problematic family relations. Thus a rigidly organized family would produce the desired high test-retest reliability, whereas a more flexible (healthy) family might not do so. Are changes in scores over a short period of time, then, indicative of family flexibility or of weakness in measurement? While this problem of interpretation exists in other types of social research, it is particularly acute in research with children (who are expected to change over time) and in research with groups of people (where there are more people who are changing over time, and where one person's change may elicit change in another)—that is, in research with families. This is not to say that interrater agreement and test-retest reliability are irrelevant in family measures, but rather that if disagreement or low stability indicators occur, one should make a sensible interpretation regarding their meaning (see Larsen & Olson, 1990, for further discussion of the possible meaning of interrater discrepancies).

Validity

In a sense, all of the issues raised in this chapter pertain to the issue of validity in family research as well. If two people (e.g., either two parents or one self-report researcher and one behavioral observer) are supposedly measuring the same construct in the same family and they come up with different descriptions, one should at least question the validity of each person's information. Further, if a measure shows little stability over time, can any one assessment be said to be a valid indicator of that trait? In addition, perhaps because family research is a relatively new field, there are few standards against which one can assess the validity of one's measure. For example, if one were trying to develop a new, short IQ test for children, the obvious standard of comparison would be one of the widely used individual IQ tests (e.g., Wechsler Intelligence Scale for Children-Revised, 1974). But where no widely used and generally accepted measure of a family construct exists (as, for example, for the constructs of enmeshment, alliance, parental warmth), it is difficult to assess the validity of new measures.

Therefore, it is particularly important that family researchers address the issues of validity. In the burgeoning field of family research, a great number of studies have recently been published. These studies are based on a wide range of theoretical frameworks and thus approach the study of families very differently, with a large number of diverse measures. Until the validity of new measures has been adequately demonstrated, it is necessary for each new user to remain skeptical and discerning about what the existing tools measure. A family-related questionnaire or observational tool may have been given a quite general name by its authors but, in fact, may measure a quite narrow, specific aspect of family process. Conversely, a measure with a specific name or description in a published study may in fact be tapping some global aspect of functioning (Grotevant, 1989). The general rules for assessing a measure's validity are the same as for any type of research, and again the reader is referred to Anastasi (1988) for a discussion of the topic.

USE OF LONGITUDINAL DESIGNS
IN FAMILY RESEARCH

In many cases, cross-sectional designs, in which data are collected at a single point in time, are quite appropriate for family researchers. The obvious advantages of cross-sectional designs over longitudinal ones (e.g., saved time, less expense, and absence of attrition) are compelling when the research question does not involve a focus on continuity, change, or predictability. Other alternatives to longitudinal designs when the question does not necessitate a focus on continuity or change are discussed in Christensen and Arrington (1987) and Achenbach (1982).

However, many family research questions do, in fact, focus on the issues of continuity, change, and predictability, and here, longitudinal designs, in which the same families are studied over time, are often the preferred strategy. Questions such as the following are best answered using longitudinal studies:

1. If fathers are nurturant to their infant daughters, are the daughters more or less likely to become independent adolescents?
2. Do husbands and wives come to dislike in each other exactly those characteristics that originally attracted them to each other?
3. After parental divorce, is an initial reaction of anger predictive of better or poorer long-term adjustment?

Longitudinal designs in family research share some problems with those in developmental research, and have some problems of their own. As is true in longitudinal research on developmental processes with children, one problem is that the appropriateness of particular measures changes with the age of the children. We might, for example, best measure "quality of mother-child relationship" through observation of play with preschoolers and through observation of a family discussion with adolescents. If we are interested in family change from the preschool to adolescent stages, we would not be able to use the same observational conditions throughout the study; this raises serious issues of comparability. Related to this issue is the problem that the manifestation of constructs is often different at different ages. For example, a "good" mother-preschooler relationship might be characterized by a high level of maternal talking and a lot of praise, whereas a "good" mother-adolescent relationship might be characterized by proportionally low levels of maternal talking and interaction of a neutral type. Thus, to the extent that longitudinal family research involves children, who are changing dramatically over the course of the study, these developmental issues are relevant.

Other issues that concern developmentalists are compounded in family research. As noted above in the discussion of reliability, even individuals are not expected to behave completely consistently from assessment to assessment; in families, we encounter this level of individual change and variability, and we encounter the phenomenon of one person's change eliciting change from other people. Deciding whether one has observed developmental change, lack of rigidity, or measurement error becomes a difficult problem.

Finally, while all longitudinal researchers, including family ones, have to cope with the problem of attrition (some people participate in the initial assessments but then drop out of the study, posing the question of whether they are different in some important way from the ones who stayed with the study throughout), family longitudinal researchers have a related problem. Even among the families who stay in a study, family constellations may change. It may be that one member refuses to participate in further assessments but the rest of the family is willing. Or, the family may have a new member: a baby, an in-law, a step-parent. Or it may have lost a member through death, divorce, or moving out. These entrances to and exits from the family change the family dramatically and in many cases should be included in the family research; however, they pose unique problems to the researcher. No standard rules about handling these problems can be offered because many complex issues about the nature of the research question and the measurement approach will determine the appropriate solution.

THE PROBLEM OF
MIXED CONCEPTUAL LEVELS
IN FAMILY RESEARCH

It should be clear by now that family research encompasses many different distinctions and strategies of study. Regardless of the design of the study, or whether the researcher chooses observational, questionnaire, or interview methods, different kinds of data may also differ as to which level of the family they concern. Cromwell and Peterson (1983) identified the following *levels* from which variables can (and, they suggest, should) be drawn. First, there is the *individual* level, a psychological and biological system that functions as the basic level of the larger family system. The next level is *dyadic,* which involves the marital, parent-child, and sibling subsystems within the family. Finally, there is the *family system* itself, which is composed of the individuals and dyads but which is presumed to be "more than the sum of its parts." Cromwell and Peterson suggest that family studies would benefit from incorporating data both from multiple types of measurement technique (e.g., behavioral observations, self-reports, clinical ratings) and from multiple levels of the family system.

Cromwell and Peterson provide a provocative case illustration of their approach using the Smiths, a family with three children, including an adolescent son who has a behavior problem. In their multisystem, multimethod assessment of the Smith family, Cromwell and Peterson administered the Minnesota Multiphasic Personality Inventory (MMPI) to the adolescent to determine his individual personality profile. They also administered several self-report measures to the mother and father about their relationship, and conducted actual observations of the couple interacting in a discussion of issues of responsibility for marital conflict. Descriptions of the couple gleaned from the different self-report measures were compared to assess convergence across measures, and descriptions of the dyad during the observation were compared with information from the self-reports to assess convergence across methods. Cromwell and Peterson observed the entire family working together for 30 minutes on a family interaction game. They also asked all members of the family to complete the Family Adaptabiity and Cohesion Evaluation Scales (FACES), a self-report measure about the family. Finally, the family participated in a family sculpture task in which family members place figurines of family members on a board in a way that represents their view of the relationship structure in the family. First, in separate rooms, individual family members each depicted the "real" and ideal family relationships, as they saw them. Then, the family worked together to depict a family consensus on real and ideal family relationships. Thus, in assessing this family, Cromwell and Peterson focused on the individual (the adolescent's MMPI), the marital (the mother's and father's reports about their relationship and the dyadic observation), and the family system (the family interaction game, the FACES, and family sculpture) levels of construct.

This case study also serves as an excellent example of yet another important dimension of family research, the differences among levels of construct, assessment, and variable formation. Each of these levels can be addressed from the individual, subsystem, or whole-family point of view. Much family research involves constructs, assessment, and variable formation at different levels. The result can be a substantial gain in information about the family (Cromwell & Peterson, 1983), but also can lead to confusion about measurement and its meaning. (See Bell & Bell [1989] and Christensen & Arrington [1987] for slightly different categorizations of these factors; and Ransom, Fisher, Phillips, Kokes, & Weiss [1990] for a more detailed system for categorizing data representing family characteristics, data generated by individuals not interacting with other family members, and data generated during family interaction.)

Level of construct refers to the level (individual, subsystem, or family) of the concept measured by the assessment tool; that is, if the measure (whether self-report or observational, based on individual or group behavior) presumably describes the whole family (e.g., the FACES, even though it was completed by individuals), the level of construct is a family one. If it presumably describes a dyad (e.g., the marital observational measure of responsibility for conflict), it is a dyadic one. And if it presumably measures an individual construct (e.g., personality structure), the level of construct is individual.

The *level of assessment* is determined by which unit of the family was actually assessed, regardless of the topic of the assessment. With self-report data, the level of assessment is usually individual, because it is an individual who fills out the questionnaire or answers the interview questions. In observational research, level of assessment refers to whose behavior (the individual, the dyad, or the family) was coded. In the Smith family, the MMPI, the mother's and father's self-reports about the marriage, the FACES, and the individually completed family sculptures were all individual-level assessments because the measures were all from individual people. Granted, in some cases the individuals were reporting on a subsystem or family, but the assessment was done individually. Assessment of the Smiths was conducted at other levels as well. Based on observations of marital and family interactions, the Smith couple were described as having a strong coalition with each other. This is a dimension that cannot belong to one person, and was derived from observation of the pair. Thus this is an example of assessment at the dyadic level. Other descriptors were more specifically about the entire family (e.g., they were "task-oriented" and "closed to negotiation"). These are examples of family-level assessment. Note that family researchers occasionally encounter trouble when trying to code a dimension at the dyadic or family level when the members of the dyad/family differ from each other on the dimension (e.g., what is a couple's marital satisfaction level if the husband seems happily married and the wife does not?). Researchers must be careful not to choose dyadic/family-level dimensions that are not conceptually dyadic/family-wide; otherwise, they force coders to make implicit decisions about how to weight individuals' input into the score. Making explicit decisions about individuals' scores should occur instead at the step of variable formation.

The *level of variable formation* refers to the level at which measures are used in coding or statistical analyses. While variable formation can, of course, be at the same level as that of assessment, individually or dyadically collected data can be used to form variables at a higher level. For example, in considering the information presented by the Smiths in response to the marital relationship questionnaires, the authors focused on topics on which there was couple disagreement. High dyadic disagreement, then, was coded on the basis of two individual reports, forming a dyadic variable from individual assessments. Observationally, the behavior of Mr. and Mrs. Smith during the couple observation was coded separately (e.g., whether each person changed his/her arguing position to agree with the other, who read instructions to whom how many times), but the behavior of both members was considered only in relation to each other; that is, both members of the couple frequently changed their arguing position, showed little disagreement with each other, and laughed a lot. The authors report this as shared, or mutual "conflict avoidance." The fact that the husband acted more as a leader than the wife was used as information, not about his leadership behavior, but as information about their role structure vis-à-vis each other. Thus, again, individual behavior was used to form a dyadic variable. In Chapter 6, we present a discussion of the various methods of combining individual scores for analyses at more complex levels (see also Fisher, Kokes, Ransom, Phillips, & Rudd, 1985).

Use of Variables of Differing Levels in Data Analysis and Interpretation

Note that once variables are formed based on data derived from individual, dyadic, or whole family measurement, the research question asked in the final statistical analysis may involve different levels of variables. One might ask how adolescents with different MMPI profiles (individual construct, assessment, and variable formation) interact with families that differ in parental marital satisfaction and family cohesion. Marital satisfaction and family cohesion refer to dyadic and family levels of construct, respectively; they may be assessed, and the variables formed, in a number of ways: through self-report or overall rating of interactions. That these analyses involve mixed levels of construct, assessment, and variable formation is not problematic statistically, but should be kept in mind in the interpretation of results. For example, it is important not to attribute a characteristic measured at the family level to an individual in the family—that is, just because a whole family is judged to be "flexible" does not mean that all its members are "flexible" in the individual sense of the term; perhaps out of the context of the family, an individual member may be quite rigid.

CONCLUSION

At every step of the research planning endeavor (idea generation, model development, and construct measurement) family researchers face both generic issues, common to other traditional social science researchers, and problems that are specific to them. Systemic theories have influenced not only our conceptualization of families but our notions of how to conduct research as well. Thus family researchers' solutions to their corpus of research problems are likely to influence the development of research methods in other areas of social science as well.

EXERCISES

1. Feldman, Wentzel, and Gehring (1989) report results of a study of the views of parents and sixth-grade boys regarding family cohesion and power. A number of interesting issues about intrafamilial agreement and agreement between self-report and observation methods are raised in this article. In addition, the measures administered and the methods used to combine data within families provide an excellent example of varying levels of construct, assessment, and variable formation. Reading this article will give you an idea of how researchers are currently addressing these concerns. Try labeling the level of construct, assessment, and variable formation for all the measures reported in the study.

2. Bell, Cornwell, and Bell (1983) report the use of a Global Coding Scheme to capture some general aspects of family functioning. Three of the construct measures were:

   a. leadership structure (from flexible to rigid)
   b. clarity (not intensity) of disclosure of feelings (from vague to clear)
   c. power hierarchy (rank order of family members in terms of who has the most influence over what happens in the family)

   Along with the rest of your class, decide on a commonly known family to rate. This could be a family in a novel, a TV family, a family depicted in a recent movie, or a real family known to all members of the class. Develop a way of assessing these three dimensions described above. Everyone in the class should then rate the family along the three dimensions. Answer the following questions:

   a. How good was the interjudge reliability across class members? How do you understand the reasons for any lack of agreement you found? Was it due to using differing information about the family? Differences in rater's standards of flexibility, clarity, or leadership? Measurement error?
   b. How might you go about establishing the validity of these ratings?

RECOMMENDED READING

Christensen, A., & Arrington, A. (1987). Research issues and strategies. In T. Jacob (Ed.), *Family interaction and psychopathology: Theories, methods, and findings* (pp. 259-296). New York: Plenum.

Cromwell, R. E., & Peterson, G. W. (1983). Multisystem-multimethod family assessment in clinical contexts. *Family Process, 22,* 147-163.

Grotevant, H. D. (1989). The role of theory in guiding family assessment. *Journal of Family Psychology, 3*(2), 104-117.

Olson, D. H. (1977). Insiders' and outsiders' views of relationships: Research and strategies. In G. Levinger & H. Raush (Eds.), *Close relationships* (pp. 115-136). Amherst: University of Massachusetts Press.

3

Self-Report Measures

Many family researchers believe that the most interesting questions about the family can be answered only through the use of observational measures—so that we can see what family members actually do in relation to each other, and not just what they say they do. There are many questions we can ask about families, however, that necessitate the use of self-report information. There is some information we can get only by asking family members directly. For example, each of the following variables is information that cannot be obtained by observing behavior but is available through self-report:

- an only child's feelings about not having siblings
- a husband's evaluation of his wife's parenting behavior
- family members' views on how close they are as a family

In family research, self-report measures can be particularly useful for obtaining measures of what Huston and Robins (1982) call "subjective conditions" and "subjective events." Subjective events are the individuals' momentary ideas, thoughts, and emotions—all of which are not directly observable. Subjective conditions are the relatively stable attitudes, attributes, and beliefs about either the partner or the relationship that arise, at least in part, out of the interaction of individuals engaged in close relationships. Subjective events and subjective conditions are contrasted with interpersonal events, which are observable behaviors, and relationship properties, which are recurrent patterns of interpersonal or subjective events.

Huston and Robins note that researchers sometimes use methods to measure relationship properties, particularly self-report measures, that are better suited to measuring subjective conditions. They suggest that in order to assess interpersonal events, some sort of observation, with concurrent recording, is the method of choice, except when the events of interest do not occur frequently enough to be captured by observational methods. In order to assess subjective conditions, the most straightforward method, and the one least subject to bias, they suggest, involves asking the participant to provide a rating or characterization of the subjective condition of interest. While concurrent reporting of the subjective condition is better than retrospective reporting, letters, diaries, and biographies can be useful sources of information about the subjective conditions that characterized particular close relationships. (See Chapter 5 for further discussion of the use of available materials in family research.)

Given that subjective conditions are probably as important to family relationships as interpersonal events, the question becomes what kinds of subjective conditions are of most interest in family research. Certainly, some important questions involve one family member's beliefs or feelings about the behaviors, beliefs, and feelings of another family member. If you hypothesized that mothers are more likely to contravene fathers when they think the fathers are too authoritarian in their child-rearing techniques, then you would need to assess the views or perceptions of the mothers concerning the fathers' child-rearing techniques. Perceptions fall under the rubric of subjective conditions, amenable to self-report methodology rather than being interpersonal events. Mothers' contravening behavior vis-à-vis fathers, by contrast, would be an interpersonal event that could be observed directly.

Self-reports can also be useful for eliciting the individual's perspective on some aspect of family life; for example, whether the family spends enough time together, the way decisions get made, or whether one's own parents are the most reactionary ones on the planet. Similarly, self-reports can be used to find out how individuals experience various aspects of family life; for example, the amount of closeness or distance they feel being expressed by other family members or the extent to which they believe their own views are respected by others.

While typically completed by individual family members, self-report measures can be used to assess family dyads or triads, the entire nuclear family, or even the extended family rather than just the individual's personal experience, recollections, and feelings. Researchers using observational techniques to study the family must necessarily rely on their own "outsider" interpretations to make sense of what they see or impose constructions on the behavior that has been recorded. Self-report techniques, by contrast, provide an "insider" view of the family and family functioning, and this view can be applied to particular dyads within the family or to the family system as a whole.

There are also pragmatic reasons for using self-report methods, and such pragmatic decisions are appropriate as long as the investigator is interested in subjective conditions rather than interpersonal events or relationship properties. For example, it is typically much less expensive to administer questionnaires, either through the mail, over the phone, or in person, or to interview family members than to observe them interacting. Researchers relying on behavioral techniques usually want a permanent record of the interaction, such as a videotape or audiotape. Such recording devices add to the costs of a project already made expensive by the demands of observing families one at a time, whether in their homes or in a university laboratory. Coding such interactional data is also extremely expensive and time consuming (see Chapter 4) but not necessarily essential to every question one might have about families. Self-report surveys also have the advantage of anonymity. If you are interested in such issues as family violence, you may be just as likely to get useful information by mailing anonymous surveys to people's homes and supplying stamped, addressed return envelopes as by asking families to allow you to observe and record the disciplinary behavior of the parents.

ISSUES IN THE USE
OF SELF-REPORT MEASURES

There are also a number of problems and limitations that must be considered if one is to rely on self-report measures. For example, self-report measures are vulnerable to a variety of distortions and biases. Thus the self-report researcher must ask, for example, what can be done to encourage subjects to present their views and values honestly rather than try to present themselves in a positive light. Can questions be worded in such a way so as to minimize various kinds of response bias, such as agreeing with every statement, disagreeing with them all (yea-saying and nay-saying), or always avoiding the more extreme scores on a rating scale and "hugging the middle?" While it is often appropriate to use self-report approaches, the limitations of these measures must be addressed and attempts to offset these limitations must be made. Fortunately, there are numerous books available that address such issues (e.g., see Fowler, 1989).

Type of Item: Global or Specific?

There are actually a variety of different types of self-report measures, each with its own advantages and disadvantages, which the researcher needs to consider in relation to the particular research questions being asked. For example, items in self-report measures can vary in the extent to which they refer to highly global evaluations or to specific behaviors and events. For example, family members could be asked to agree or disagree with such broad statements as:

* In our family, we all get along very well.
* My parents are very understanding.
* I come from a warm and caring family.

While such global evaluations can yield some very useful data in family research, they can be contaminated by response sets, such as social desirability (the tendency to describe oneself as possessing characteristics that are valued in one's culture). Consequently, there is a push within the field to develop various kinds of approaches that focus on more specific behaviors. Some investigators have developed a behavioral report approach in which they ask family members to report on various events and behaviors that occurred within a specified time period. If you wanted to use a behavioral report approach to issues of conflict resolution in marital couples, you might ask husbands and wives to agree or disagree with such statements as the following:

* In the past 12 hours . . .
  my spouse and I had a disagreement over a minor issue.
  my spouse and I had a disagreement over a major issue.
  I yelled at my spouse.
  my spouse yelled at me.
  I listened to my spouse's point of view.
  my spouse listened to my point of view.

While such items are not necessarily entirely safeguarded from tendencies toward social desirability, they have the virtue of being focused on rather specific behaviors, leaving less to the interpretation of the respondent.

Format: Open Ended or Closed?

Not all self-report approaches are of the limited response type illustrated above, where people are asked to agree or disagree with statements, or to rate items for how well they describe the self or other family members. Questionnaires typically have this closed-ended, objective format, but interviews, another form of self-report, are more often open

---

BOX 3.1
Guidelines for Writing Self-Report Items
(and Examples of Some Failures)

1. All questions should be clear and unambiguous.
   Failure: How is your family?
2. The vocabulary used in the items should be appropriate to the educational level and experience of your respondents.
   Failure: I am interested in learning about families. Would you call your family enmeshed or disengaged?
3. The questions should not demand information your respondents do not have.
   Failure: How do you think your spouse *really* feels, deep down inside, about the way you make love?
4. You should present a clear frame of reference for the questions so that your subjects interpret the questions the way you do, or be prepared to elicit *their* frame of reference.
   Failure: I am interested in families. So, what is your spouse like? (The respondent has no idea whether you are interested in the partner's sex role, way of dealing with conflict, feelings about the marriage, and so forth.)
5. Focus each item on a single idea rather than touch on separate problems that might or might not evoke similar responses.
   Failure: Would you say you and your spouse have problems in communicating or do you have a pretty good marriage?

---

ended, calling for people to respond to questions in their own words. Although open-ended questionnaires allow for potentially more relevant information, they are more costly to administer because they involve a one-to-one dialogue between interviewer and respondent.

If you are interested in conflict resolution and wish to obtain rich, detailed data, you might ask family members such questions as the following:

- What types of issues lead to disagreements within your family?
- Typically, how do such disagreements get handled?
- Give me an example of some disagreement among family members that really got handled well.

Box 3.1 provides a brief summary of guidelines for developing self-report measures, particularly of the closed-ended type, and examples of items that do not adhere to the guidelines. Issues in coding open-ended material are discussed in greater detail below.

CODING OPEN-ENDED VERBAL MATERIAL

Interviews have the advantage of richness of detail and reliance on the respondents' own words, but unless the researcher wishes to keep responses in a purely qualitative form, they need to be coded—that is, the investigator must find some way of making the qualitative verbal information quantitative so that it can be analyzed statistically. Coding involves categorizing the verbal material in ways that capture the variables of interest. When interviews have been audiotaped (like videotapes of behavioral interactions), they provide a permanent record that can be coded again and again by investigators with different interests and perspectives.

Suppose, for example, that David and Natalie, the husband and wife introduced in Chapter 1, gave the answers found in Box 3.2 when each was interviewed separately by an investigator who said, "I am interested in how spouses feel about issues of separateness and togetherness. How do you feel when your spouse wants to do something without you? How does your spouse feel when you want to do something without him/her? Please give me some specific examples."

Here is some fairly detailed and credible information about issues of togetherness and separateness in one married couple. David and Nancy, like other intimate partners, may have discrepant ideas about the meaning of togetherness and separateness within a marriage, the extent to which doing things together and separately is important to the marriage, the extent to which one can love one's partner but still want private time, and other issues. But suppose you are working within a conceptual framework in which separateness is not considered the opposite of togetherness, and both shared and independent activities are seen as contributing to a healthy marriage. Suppose also that you have interviewed a number of couples and are addressing the following questions:

1. To what extent do husbands and wives have similar views of the extent to which they need both separate and shared activities?
2. To what extent is consensus concerning separate and shared activities associated with a measure of marital adjustment?

If you had interviewed Nancy and David as well as other couples, you might want to ask some additional questions to probe for more detail about their feelings, or to ask for some additional examples. But

---

BOX 3.2
Open-Ended Responses From David and Nancy

David: "Well, Nancy is much bigger on the togetherness stuff than I am. I guess she's a typical woman. We both work and she's away a lot, so we really don't have much time to do things together. I spend a lot of time with my daughter during the week, so I like to go out with the guys for a beer on Friday nights. Usually Nancy is pretty good about that, but she starts complaining when she feels neglected. She takes an art class on Saturday and of course I don't mind her fooling around with her paints if she wants, but I wish she could take the class on Friday nights when I'm out. I think she should be there when I'm home. Sometimes she wants to take in a movie with some of her friends."

Nancy: "It's seems as though mostly everything we do is separate. When we're both at home, which isn't all that much, he likes to watch the sports channel on TV and I usually read or work on reports. He goes out with the boys every Friday night, and that's the only night it's O.K. for me to go out. I love to go to the movies with my friends and we like to go Sunday night because it's not so crowded, but he complains if I'm not at home to make his supper and bring him a snack. He also doesn't like my seeing friends just to talk, because he's sure we gossip about him. It wouldn't be so bad if he wanted to go out with me once in awhile but he's always too tired or there's some game he doesn't want to miss."

---

even without further probing, you have learned some important things about togetherness and separateness in this couple. So, what would you do with the information? How would you code their responses?

Typically, investigators have a driving conceptual framework that informs both the questions they ask and their preliminary plans for coding the replies. It is useful for them to have at least a rough coding scheme in mind, or they may later find that they have not asked the very questions that are most essential to obtaining replies that are analyzable and interpretable within their theoretical framework. Researchers analyzing the responses you just read might have adopted any of the

following strategies, depending on their particular views on togetherness and separateness, and the particular questions they were asking:

1. applying 7-point rating scales (with 1 being low and 7 being high) to rate
   the extent to which each respondent seems to value or be concerned with
   his or her own separateness, other's separateness, his or her own togetherness, other's togetherness;
2. categorizing each respondent into one of two groups: (a) primarily concerned with achieving greater togetherness, or (b) primarily concerned
   with achieving greater separateness;
3. giving each respondent a score of 1 (satisfied) or 0 (dissatisfied) on each
   of the following dimensions: (a) satisfaction with degree of separateness
   characterizing the spousal interaction, and (b) satisfaction with degree of
   togetherness characterizing the spousal interaction.

Obviously, there are other ways to analyze the material in the quotes
by David and Nancy as well, and you may want to think of some
approaches that would be interesting. Whatever strategy is chosen, you
would have to develop criteria and guidelines so that independent
scorers would have an adequate basis for making reliable (consistent)
judgments. Right now, if you and a friend both tried to score David and
Nancy according to any of the scoring suggestions mentioned above,
you might find yourselves quickly engaged in a heated debate. Although
debates between scorers can happen even when investigators have
devoted years to developing scoring guidelines, a good, clear detailed
set of guidelines is essential to the process of training reliable coders
(i.e., coders whose scores are consistent with each other when they have
scored the same material by the same guidelines).

Look at the sample quotes again. If you were going to score David
and Nancy (and other husbands and wives answering the same question)
on the extent to which they are preoccupied with issues of separateness
as compared to issues of togetherness, what else would you want
besides clear coding guidelines? Probably you would like a larger
sample of relevant information from each respondent. Whether one is
doing a self-report study, an observational study or a secondary analysis
of data, an important question is always whether one has an adequate
sample of the views or behaviors of interest to obtain reliable and valid
data.

ADVANTAGES AND DISADVANTAGES
OF DIFFERENT TYPES OF SELF-REPORTS

Both the open-ended and closed-ended types of self-report measures have their own particular advantages and disadvantages. The closed-ended, fixed-response (e.g., true-false, multiple-choice) format is particularly useful in large surveys. If you are interested in the ways family members solve conflicts, and want to be able to generalize findings to a variety of groups around the country, then a fixed-response format, of the type used by Murray Straus and his colleagues from the University of New Hampshire to assess methods of conflict resolution (e.g., Straus, 1979), is particularly valuable. Instruments of the fixed response variety can be duplicated and distributed to a large number of people relatively inexpensively, and scoring is completely objective. Thus, external validity (the extent to which findings from a sample can be generalized) is relatively easy to establish, and there are no problems of intercoder reliability. On the other hand, such survey instruments may have problems of construct validity—that is, the investigator cannot assume that the responses necessarily reflect the issues the investigator intended to assess. What if most of the people who received, completed, and returned a mailed survey misunderstood one of the questions and this affected everybody's score in a misleading way? The investigators might not have any way of realizing what had happened and thus would be likely to misinterpret the scores derived from the surveys.

Open-ended response formats, of the type commonly found in interviews, have the advantage of providing opportunities for the interviewer to clarify misunderstandings and, if necessary, to revise the interview to reduce the likelihood of misunderstandings. Moreover, because the interviewer can probe for additional information, as necessary, to assess a construct fully, open-ended interviews are less likely to be subject to the problems of construct validity that affect large-scale self-administered surveys. On the other hand, because open-ended interviews are costly to administer and score, they frequently are used with small available samples and may be subject to problems of external validity. A researcher might find that a group of well-educated, middle-class Boston husbands are higher in warmth and nurturance than their wives, and that their degree of warmth and nurturance is related to their wives' marital satisfaction, but it would be unacceptable to assume either that all husbands are warmer and more nurturant than their wives, or that there will always be the same degree of association between husbands' nurturance and wives' marital satisfaction. Open-ended response formats also have the disadvantage that intercoder reliability must be established as well as being subject to interviewer bias.

SOURCES OF AVAILABLE MEASURES

With a little bit of good detective work, you may find that an instrument of known reliability and validity has already been developed that is well suited for investigating a problem of interest to you. Certainly, if you can find an adequate instrument, it will free you of the laborious and time-consuming task of developing your own measure, pilot-testing it, administering it to a normative sample (i.e., a sample selected to represent the population for which the measure is designed to be used), and establishing its reliability and validity.

So, where do you start your detective work? A survey of the literature in your area of interest may help uncover both published and unpublished self-report measures and provide some relevant information about reliability and validity. At the end of this chapter, we suggest some additional references that were useful in the preparation of the following summary and that should be of value to the interested reader. In the remainder of this chapter, we provide a brief description of some sample self-report instruments that have been used in the study of family relationships. We have not tried to be exhaustive in our review, but merely to give the reader an idea of the range of instruments available and a few of the pros and cons of using them. We start with measures of dyadic functioning (parent-child and spousal relations), and then consider approaches directed more at family systems.

Parent-Child Relations

Child Abuse Potential Inventory. Following a literature review to identify personality traits characteristic of individuals who abuse or neglect children, Milner and Wimberley (1979) constructed a measure that they hoped could provide a quick, client-administered screening device for assessing an individual's potential for child abuse. A preliminary version of the Child Abuse Potential Inventory was administered to 19 abusing and 19 matched nonabusing parents, and an item analysis was conducted to identify items distinguishing between the groups. The final 160 items of the measure includes seven abuse scales (Abuse, Distress, Rigidity, Unhappiness, Problems with Child and Self, Problems with Family, and Problems from Others), three validity scales (a lie scale, a random response scale, and an inconsistency scale), and several filler items—all of which are responded to in an "agree/disagree" format.

Milner (1986) indicates that internal consistency estimates range from .50 to .90 for the various subscales, while split-half reliabilities are in the .90s. Test-retest reliabilities range from the low .90s following a 1-week interval to .75 after a 3-month interval. Information about content, construct, and criterion-related validity can be found in the manual (Milner, 1986). In general, support for the validity of the measure comes from studies indicating that it can be used to differentiate abusing from nonabusing parents. Nevertheless, one problem with the Milner measure is the danger of overinterpretation of "potential" for child abuse. Although the measure has successfully differentiated samples of abusing parents from nonabusers, it is not clear how many people may score high on the inventory without being abusive. In other words, while high scores on the inventory as a whole may be found in some samples of abusive parents, it is not clear to what extent the measure may be susceptible to both false positives and false negatives as a diagnostic instrument.

Block Child Rearing Practices Report. The Child Rearing Practices Report (CRPR) was developed by Jeanne Block (1966) to assess parental socialization behaviors from the perspective of either parents or their children. The original CRPR consisted of two sets of 91 statements each, one for mothers' child-rearing behaviors and one for fathers' behaviors. The items were originally developed to be administered in a semistructured Q-sort format, wherein items are typed on separate cards that subjects sort into a designated number of piles according to how well the statements describe them. The items can also be presented in other formats—for example, as 7-point scales on which respondents rate the extent to which the behavior was or was not characteristic of the parent when the respondent was a child (e.g., Costos, 1986). Items such as "My mother wanted me to solve problems on my own" are typical of the measure.

Block (1973) has reported relatively high levels of test-retest reliability for the CRPR measure across intervals up to 3 years. Roberts, Block, and Block (1984) report substantial continuity in child-rearing orientations (e.g., Authoritarian Control, Emphasis on Achievement, and Encouraging Openness to Experience). Other investigators who created scales for mutuality-oriented and control-oriented practices (Sklover, White, & Wenar, 1988) and parental agency and communion (Costos, 1986) have reported adequate internal consistency for these scales (with alphas ranging from .66 to .92).

While the instrument is time consuming for respondents to complete, especially when it is administered in the Q-sort format, and requires a sixth-grade-level reading ability, it has a number of advantages. For example, the Q-sort format mitigates the effects of response bias. Moreover, since the measure has been used in many different studies and translated into several languages, it can be used for making cross-cultural comparisons of child-rearing attitudes and their correlates.

Spousal Relationships: Marital Adjustment and Quality

Within the family studies literature, there has been a long-standing interest in the concept of marital adjustment. Unfortunately, as Spanier and Cole pointed out in 1976, consensus concerning the meaning of the concept is notable for its absence. Spanier and Cole note that the problem with marital adjustment is like the problem with love—everybody "knows" what the term means until it comes to the development of an operational definition. Basically, measures of adjustment seem to focus on issues presumed to be essential to a harmonious and well-adjusted relationship.

Locke-Wallace Marital Adjustment Scales. The Locke-Wallace Marital Adjustment scales (Locke & Wallace, 1959) have been widely used to provide a global measure of marital adjustment, defined by Locke and Wallace as the "accommodation of a husband and wife to each other at a given time" (p. 251). Their 15-item fixed-response marital adjustment test consists of 1 item that asks respondents to indicate on a 7-point scale the degree of happiness they experience in their marriage, as well as 8 items concerning the extent of spousal agreement on such issues as finances, recreation, and philosophy of life, and 6 items posing such questions as who gives in when a disagreement occurs and how the couple uses leisure time.

Locke and Wallace report high internal consistency for the marital adjustment test, as well as satisfactory discrimination of a sample of maladjusted couples from a sample of well-adjusted couples. However, there is evidence that Locke-Wallace test scores are contaminated by respondents' tendencies to distort the appraisal of their marriage in a socially desirable direction. Moreover, it has been argued (Spanier, 1973) that the test assesses individual adjustment to the marriage rather than the marriage relationship itself. Perhaps a bigger problem is that the scale includes both the kind of individual-level items that Huston and Robins (1982) describe as measuring subjective conditions (e.g., Do you ever wish you had not married?) and more dyadic items focusing more on relationship properties (e.g, When disagreements arise, they usually result in: husband giving in, wife giving in, or agreement by mutual give and take?). Despite such limitations, many of the items in the measure still see wide use, partly because they have been incorporated into Graham Spanier's popular measure of dyadic adjustment.

Spanier Dyadic Adjustment Scale. Spanier and Cole (1976) were critical of global measures of marital adjustment, such as the Locke-Wallace scales, on the grounds that such approaches paid little attention to the distinctions among such concepts as satisfaction, happiness, stability, success, and adjustment, and that they assessed adjustment as a qualitative state rather than as a process. According to Spanier and Cole, marital adjustment is a process, the outcome of which is determined by such issues as degree of troublesome marital differences, interspousal tensions and personal anxiety, marital satisfaction, dyadic cohesion, and consensus on important matters.

Spanier (1976) reported on the development of the Dyadic Adjustment Scale, a 32-item self-report scale designed for use with either married or unmarried cohabiting couples. The measure consists of four subscales (dyadic satisfaction, dyadic cohesion, dyadic consensus, and affectional expression) that were, according to Spanier, empirically verified through factor analysis and characterized by high internal consistency. Spanier presents evidence in support of the content, criterion-related, and construct validity of the measure.

While the Dyadic Adjustment Scale has had wide use in marriage and family research, it does have a number of limitations. While Spanier claims that the separate dimensions have been empirically verified, there is evidence that the scale is really unidimensional (Carmines & Zeller, 1979). Problems also arise because the separate scales differ in length and response format. Finally, like the Locke-Wallace Inventory, the measure combines individually and dyadically oriented items in a way that may have unknown effects on the results.

Waring Intimacy Questionnaire. The Waring Intimacy Questionnaire (Waring & Reddon, 1983). was developed in accordance with the theoretical position that interpersonal dyadic relationships can be defined by three relatively independent dimensions: boundary, process, and intimacy. Waring and associates (e.g., Waring, McElrath, Mitchell, & Derry, 1981) hold that intimacy is the primary dimension determining marital adjustment.

The Waring Intimacy Questionnaire consists of 8 scales designed to assess conceptually derived dimensions of marital intimacy: conflict resolution, affection, cohesion, sexuality, identity, compatibility, autonomy, and expressiveness. Items are presented in a true-false format, and are constructed to avoid an acquiescence bias. Statistical analyses have been conducted to identify the 40 most efficient items from the subscales, and these 40 items can be used to derive a global measure of intimacy. Waring and associates administer a social desirability scale along with the intimacy scales, and suggest that users of the intimacy questionnaire subtract the social desirability score from the total intimacy score.

A number of questions can be raised about the reliability and validity of the Waring scales. For example, some of the subscales appear to be quite limited in internal consistency, which in turn imposes limitations on both reliability and validity. It is interesting that the autonomy subscale, which is directed at the couples' orientation to interpersonal relationships outside the marriage, including parents, children, and friends, is, of all the subscales, lowest in internal consistency and the least well predicted by a measure of self-disclosure (Waring & Chelune, 1983).

White Intimacy Maturity Interview. While most of the available instruments for assessing family systems and subsystems are closed-ended in format, there are open-ended measures with detailed coding systems. For example, White and her associates (e.g., White et al., 1986; White, Speisman, Costos, & Smith, 1987; White, Houlihan, Speisman, & Costos, 1990) have developed a semistructured interview and scoring manual (White, Speisman, Costos, Jackson, & Bartis, in press) for determining individuals' levels of maturity within their closest relationships. Questions (e.g., What is your view of your partner? What is your partner's view of you? How do you show caring toward each other? How do disagreements get handled?) cover five areas of the relationship: orientation (to the other and the relationship), caring/concern, communication, commitment, and sex. The intimacy maturity scoring manual is used to code responses to the open-ended interview questions into three broad levels of intimacy maturity: self-focused, role-focused, and individuated-connected. Each of these levels has two substages. With the inclusion of transitional stages, the whole system converts into an 11-point scale. White et al. (1986) report average intercoder reliability coefficients of .65 among three independent raters on the five scales of the intimacy maturity interview; the average correlation between each scorer's original score and the final score arrived at after discussion was .80. Construct validity information is reported for the interview and scoring system in White et al. (1986) and White et al. (in press). Because of the richness of the interview, it has also proven amenable to scoring for other constructs—for example, empathy (Monahan, 1989), narcissism (Layton, 1988), intimacy processes (Paul, 1989), and interpersonal development (Bar-Yam Hassam, 1989). As with any one-on-one interview approach, the intimacy maturity interview is more costly to use than self-administered and objectively scored questionnaires, but it provides a wealth of rich qualitative data about close dyadic relationships and is amenable to the derivation of quantitative scores.

Peterson Interaction Record. Peterson (1979) developed the Interaction Record as a method of studying interaction processes in interpersonal relationships. The fundamental unit of an interaction process is, according to Peterson, an *interaction sequence,* which he defines as beginning when an act by one participant in a relationship is followed by contingent action on the part of the other, and continuing as long as reciprocal contingency prevails in the ensuing interaction. Couples using the interaction form are instructed to describe the most important interaction they had that day. Using their own words, and describing the interaction from their individual viewpoints, the partners are instructed to describe the conditions under which the exchange took place, how the interaction started, and what happened then.

Peterson has developed a coding system to analyze the written reports provided by couples to describe their most important interactions. He begins by categorizing the interaction into major "moves" (e.g., husband embraces wife, wife says she does not want to cuddle, husband withdraws and goes to sleep). He then infers an interpersonal meaning, or message, from each act. These messages fall into three categories: affect (I hate you), construal (Now I'm sure you understand me), and expectations (Now I think you'll leave me alone). From his analyses, Peterson identified several types of affect, construal, and expectation characterizing important interactions, most of which served effectively to distinguish among disturbed, average, and satisfied couples.

Peterson believes that his method provides a useful approach to acquiring data on "living interactions" that are difficult to describe by other means. He suggests that the very subjectivity of the reports allows researchers to study covert processes as well as overt behavior, but without some of the problems of more traditional self-report techniques. An expansion of this technique can be found in the work of Huston, Robins, Atkinson, and McHale (1987), who have also developed a behavioral self-report procedure to use with married couples. However, in contrast with Peterson's approach, Huston and colleagues developed a telephone interview procedure to obtain reports on behaviors of interest. These telephone interviews, scheduled in advance, sample five domains of activity identified as important to the marital relationship: household tasks, leisure activities, positive and negative interactions, conflict episodes, and conversations with the spouse and others. Information about these activity domains can be summarized to provide measures of companionship, involvement with others, and marital role performance. Research using the method (Huston et al., 1987) has generated information about behavioral changes in the first year of marriage, forces affecting the division of household tasks, and forces affecting parental roles with infants. While the method is extremely time consuming, Huston and colleagues note that their ability to break down a construct, such as division of labor, into its components (i.e., specific activities of spouses) and then aggregate the specific data in a variety of ways is perhaps the greatest methodological advantage of collecting data at the level of specific events.

Comments on Dyadic Measures

While many family researchers believe we must move beyond individual measures and assess dyads and whole families if we are truly to understand close relationships and dyadic and systemic interactions, dyadic measures have their own particular problems and limitations that must be addressed. Each of the measures described above yields a score for the individual respondent. While scores from participants in a relationship can be combined in various ways to create a dyadic score (see Chapter 6), most of the measures provide views or evaluations of the relationship rather than direct interactional data of the sort that can be obtained with observational methods. Thus it is important to remember that even if we combine partners' scores on, for example, Spanier's Dyadic Adjustment Scales, the scores represent partners' characterizations of their communication rather than their communication behavior per se.

Self-Reports of Family System Functioning

Family Environment Scale. The Family Environment Scale (Moos, 1974; Moos & Moos, 1981) was one of the first self-report measures developed to assess the family as a system. The measure consists of 10 subscales designed to assess the following three broad domains of family functioning: (a) relationship dimensions (cohesion, expressiveness, and conflict); (b) personal growth dimensions (independence, achievement orientation, intellectual-cultural orientation, active-recreational orientation, and moral-religious emphasis); and (c) systems maintenance dimensions (organization and control).

The 90-item Family Environment Scale comes in three forms: *Form R,* the Real Form, which assesses individuals' perceptions of their family environments; *Form E,* the Expectations Form, which assesses individual expectations about family settings; and *Form I,* the Ideal Form, which is directed at conceptions of ideal family environments. There is considerable evidence supporting the reliability and validity of the scales (Moos & Moos, 1981; Fowler, 1982a, 1982b). For example, alpha coefficients ranging from .61 to .78 suggest adequate internal consistency, and data from more than 200 studies provide construct validation for the measure (Moos & Spinrad, 1984).

There is also a children's version of the Family Environment Scale— titled, rather unambiguously, the Children's Version of the Family Environment Scale (CVFES). This 30-item multiple-choice measure consists of pictures used to assess children's perceptions of their family's social climate. Intended for children between the ages of 5 and 12 years, this measure has not yet been demonstrated to have adequate reliability and validity as an extension of the Family Environment Scale.

Family Adaptability and Cohesion Evaluation Scales. Working within their circumplex model of family functioning (see Chapter 2), Olson and his colleagues (Olson, Russell, & Sprenkle, 1979, 1983; Olson, Sprenkle, & Russell, 1979) developed the Family Adaptability and Cohesion Evaluation Scales (FACES) to assess two dimensions derived from the family therapy literature. They define family cohesion as the emotional bonding that family members have with each other, and family adaptability as the ability of the marital or family system to change its power structure. The circumplex model also identifies a third dimension, family communication, which is hypothesized to facilitate movement on the two axes defined by cohesion and adaptability.

The FACES scales are designed to permit classification of families as a function of (a) their degree of cohesion, which can range from extremely low (disengaged) through moderate or balanced (separated, connected) to extremely high (enmeshed); and (b) their degree of adaptability, which can range from extremely low (rigid) through moderate (flexible, structured) to extremely high (chaotic). Families are considered to be functioning well if they are characterized by moderate levels of cohesion and adaptability, although Olson, Russell, and Sprenkle have suggested that families that are extreme on both dimensions can function well if all members like it that way.

Validational studies (e.g., Portner, 1981; Bell, 1982) of the first FACES measure indicated that nonproblem families were more likely than clinical families to fall into the balanced range on the two scales.

FACES III (Olson, Portner, & Lavee, 1985), a more recent version of the measure, is administered in two formats: the perceived family ("How would you describe your family now?"), and the ideal family ("How would you like your family to be?"). Satisfaction with family can be computed by calculating the magnitude of the discrepancy between perceived and ideal scores. FACES III also has both a family and a couple version. Australian research (Noller & Shum, 1990) with the couple version of the measure demonstrated that FACES III was useful in discriminating between families high and low on the cohesion factors; however, a 17-item version of the scale was more reliable than the 20-item version. Olson (1990) has himself now recommended that researchers and clinicians use the 17-item version of the scale.

Normative data reveal that scores from different members of the same family can be highly discrepant, thus indicating that different members can have very different perspectives on the family system. Chapter 6 provides some guidelines for dealing with family scores in those circumstances. In addition, various forms of the FACES measure have been criticized both for the underlying conceptualization and on empirical grounds (e.g., Beavers & Voeller, 1983). Olson appears to have been responsive to these criticisms in his revisions of the measure, and it seems likely that researchers will continue to explore the usefulness of the measure and the circumplex approach.

McMaster Family Assessment Device. The McMaster Family Assessment Device (FAD) is a 60-item self-report measure designed to assess six dimensions of family functioning: problem solving, communication, roles, affective responsiveness, affective involvement, and behavior control. It also includes a general functioning scale to assess overall health versus pathology. A recent psychometric study (Kabacoff, Miller, Bishop, Epstein, & Keitner, 1990) reported alpha coefficients for the separate scales ranging from .57 (the roles scale) to .86 (the general functioning scale). A factor analysis of the 48 items not on the general functioning scale (which is assumed to be correlated with all the other scales) revealed that 44 items (92%) loaded highest on the factor they were hypothesized to represent. Moreover, a comparison of the hypothesized factor structure based on the McMaster Model of Family Functioning (MMFF) with several alternative factor models revealed that the MMFF model accounted for more variance in scores than the alternative models. The General Functioning Scale, hypothesized to be predictive of scores on all the other scales, correlated .85, .87, and .88 with the first principal component derived from the factor analyses in nonclinical, psychiatric, and medical samples, respectively.

Kabacoff and colleagues conclude that using the standard criterion of .70 for the reliability of a research instrument, six of the seven FAD scales demonstrated adequate internal reliabilities in large nonclinical, psychiatric, and medical samples. They note that the Roles scale was the sole exception, with marginal reliability in the psychiatric and medical samples (alpha = .69) and lower reliability in the nonclinical sample (.57). Moreover, the results of the confirmatory factor analyses provided support for the hypothesized structure of the instrument.

Family Assessment Measure. Skinner, Steinhauer, and Santa-Barbara (1983) developed the Family Assessment Measure (FAM) to assess family strengths and weaknesses. The measure has three subscales: a General scale, focusing on the family as a system; a Dyadic Relationships scale, measuring the relationships of specific pairs within the family; and a Self-Rating scale, which taps each member's perception of his or her functioning within the family system. The measure is derived from a process model of family functioning that emphasizes achievement of a variety of basic, developmental, and crisis tasks (Task Accomplishment) as the basic goal of the family. Fundamental to task accomplishment are role performance, communication, affective expression, involvement, control, and values and norms.

A recent version of the measure, FAM III, consists of 132 items that can be completed by all members of a family who are at least 10 to 12 years old. The General scale (50 items) is designed to assess overall health or pathology in the family from a systems perspective. It contains 7 subscales relating to the constructs in the process model (for example, task accomplishment, role performance, and communication). The Dyadic Relationship scale (42 items) focuses on relationships among specific dyads (e.g., husband-wife, mother-daughter) in the family. An overall rating of family functioning can be derived for each dyad, along with scores on 7 subscales relating to constructs in the process model. The Self-Rating scale (42 items) focuses on an individual's perception of his or her functioning in the family. An overall index can be derived, along with 7 subscale scores.

Skinner and colleagues provide evidence supporting the internal consistency of the three principal scales and the subscales of the FAM III measure. In support of validity, they report substantial negative correlations between FAM III scores and social desirability and defensiveness, as well as evidence that General scale scores differentiated problem from nonproblem families. Finally, Skinner and colleagues report only moderate correlations (mean = .36) between husbands' and wives' portrayals of their family.

Comments on Family Systems Measures

While these four family systems measures constitute a breakthrough in their focus on characteristics of families rather than characteristics of individuals, they nevertheless are limited in that they can give us only individual perceptions of the family rather than a more direct measure of actual family functioning. While one can try to create a couple or family score by such tactics as averaging the scores of different family members (see Chapter 6), there are always some problems in interpreting such combined scores, particularly given the relatively low consensus between family members concerning what their family is like. Nevertheless, despite the limitations of such measures, they provide one more avenue for attempting to understand family interactional processes from the perspective of family members.

EXERCISES

1. What's wrong with these self-report items? (see Box 3.1)
   1. Do you and your husband agree on most things or do you sometimes wish you had never gotten married?

2. Which of your children do you like the best?
3. Where does your family fit on the circumplex model?
4. How does your family compare with other families?
5. What degree of cohesion and adaptability is characteristic of your family?

2. Suppose you are interested in learning about patterns of communication between parents and adolescents. Formulate 5 to 10 questions that you could ask parents and another set that you could pose to adolescents. Have a friend use the criteria in Box 3.1 to evaluate your questions. How would you score answers to the questions? Is your measure aimed primarily at the individual, dyadic, or family systems level?

3. Several of the measures described in this chapter are available right within published articles that describe them (e.g., Spanier, 1976; Straus, 1979). Others (e.g., White et al., in press) are available from Social and Behavioral Sciences Documents, P.O. Box 9838, San Rafael, CA 94912. Most others can be obtained by writing directly to their authors; addresses are typically available in the articles describing the measures. Start to develop a collection of measures and compare them for issues covered, format, and other factors. Develop hypotheses that could be tested using one or more of these measures.

RECOMMENDED READING

Huston, T. L., & Robins, E. (1982). Conceptual and methodological issues in studying close relationships. *Journal of Marriage and the Family, 44,* 901-925.

Skinner, H. A. (1987). Self-report instruments for family assessment. In T. Jacob (Ed.), *Family interaction and psychopathology* (pp. 427-452). New York: Plenum.

4

Observational Methods

A variety of self-report measures useful in studying families were reviewed in the previous chapter. The advantages of simply asking people about the variable of interest are clear. Many researchers, however, prefer to observe families directly. Instead of asking members of a family how they get along, families are asked to talk or to do some kind of task together in front of a video camera or the researcher, and the family is coded along some dimension of "getting along-ness." This approach usually involves complicated equipment, microphones, the need for standard data collection facilities, and highly trained data collectors and coders, all of which are costly in terms of time and money. One worries whether what is observed is "what the family is really like," and whether the "essence" of the family can really be coded by outsiders who, by definition, do not know the family well. Nevertheless, there are compelling reasons to adopt this approach, at least as one component of a study of families.

THE ISSUE OF BIAS

First, unlike self-reports, observational methods do not involve asking the subjects about themselves, so a number of potential sources of bias are eliminated. In self-reports, people may have a conscious or not-so-conscious desire to portray themselves or their families differently than they really are. A husband and wife with a child who has a lot of problems, for example, may think of themselves as quite happily married ("if only Joey would shape up"), and all their family members might complete a questionnaire saying so. In observing the couple and child discuss an issue, however, it may be quite clear that there is a lot of veiled hostility between the spouses.

Distortion in self-report may be simply a matter of trying to make oneself or one's family look better or worse than they really are, but the motive need not be so devious. There are many psychological constructs of great interest to researchers to which people simply do not have access in regard to themselves. People may not know how "typical" they are, for example. In this regard, consider the question, "Do you and your sibling fight a lot?" Respondents may know roughly how they compare to their neighbors, schoolmates, or extended family, but the families in these groups are likely to be quite similar to their own family. In the example of the couple given above, the husband and wife may truly think of themselves as having no direct conflict with each other, though in fact the problem child may be providing a convenient distractor from such conflict. Direct observation of the families can provide objective information about the behavior of the members, avoiding some of these problems of bias.

While some bias problems are reduced, others may be heightened in observational methods, of course. Family members may act differently just because they know they are being observed (Haynes & Horn, 1982; Kazdin, 1982; Reid, Baldwin, Patterson, & Dishion, 1988). This alteration may be an attempt at impression management (e.g., families can try to hide their conflicts while being observed, or try to make one person look like more or less of a problem than he/she is) or may be nonspecific in nature (e.g., they may be nervous, artificial; see Pollack, Vincent, & Williams [1977]; cited in Reid et al. [1988]). Various approaches have been taken to assess the role of reactivity in affecting observations. For example, parents have been asked to make their children's behavior better than normal (to "fake good") or worse than normal (to "fake bad"). While it seems that parents of normal children can alter their children's behavior in response to these specific demands (Johnson & Lobitz, 1974), they seem better at faking bad than faking good (Lobitz & Johnson, 1975). This was especially the case for families with problem children (Reid et al., 1988). Also, children's classroom behavior has been compared in conditions when an observer was visible versus times when he or she was hidden behind a one-way mirror (Weinrott, Garrett, & Todd, 1978), and families' at-home behavior has been compared when an observer was present versus instances when he or she was absent and the behavior was recorded only by an audio recording (Johnson & Bolstad, 1975); little support was found for the impression management problem (Reid et al. 1988). In contrast, Baum, Forehand, and Zegiob (1979) concluded that parents changed their positive behavior (e.g., playing with child, giving praise) more than their negative behavior (e.g., disapproving comments) in the presence of an observer. In general, observational researchers assume that, while their presence may alter or constrain subjects' behavior, people cannot profoundly change their behavior, at least not all levels of it, just by trying to do so. A number of measures can be taken to reduce the reactivity of the observational setting (i.e., the degree to which family members alter their behavior because they are participating in a research study) or at least to measure it; these are discussed in a later section.

THE ISSUE OF WHOLE VERSUS PARTS

A second limit of self-report methods is that they are inherently individually based approaches to understanding a problem. Unless a questionnaire is completed by the whole family (in which case the process of the completion—who dominates, who gives in, who makes suggestions—is usually observed), self-reports are completed by one person. In contrast, observations allow the assessment of the whole family (or the complete couple, in marriage research) at one time. While many observational coding systems do, in fact, include coding of the behavior of one person at a time (e.g., number of criticisms that the father makes), the potential is there to characterize the whole family with just one variable (e.g., how much tension exists during the interaction).

THE ISSUE OF ACCESS

Observational studies can also provide a look at families with young children, or with disturbed members, who would not be able to report very well on themselves or their families.

THE ISSUE OF BEHAVIOR VERSUS SELF-PERCEPTION

Finally, observational methods are important because actual behavioral sequences are fundamental to many important constructs in family systems theories; the ability to measure them reliably and validly is thus critical. For example, suppose one predicts that disturbed children often get mixed messages from their parents—the parents say one thing but the nonverbal messages, like the tone of voice, degree of sarcasm, or hand gestures, say quite another. Relying on self-report would tap only one half of this important equation. Or suppose a researcher interested in marital conflict predicts that, in conflicted couples as opposed to nonconflicted couples, the verbalization of one spouse is more often followed by silence or delayed response. These conflicted spouses might correctly report on a questionnaire that few hostile remarks are exchanged between them, but their interaction pattern is, indeed, quite marked. Rogers, Millar, and Bavelas (1985) present a concise argument for the necessity of including observable, sequential, and systems-level behavioral descriptions if family research is to be truly relational and systemic.

CHOOSING A TASK FOR OBSERVATION

What should the family actually *do* in front of that video camera? Especially with older, camera-conscious children, it would be uncomfortable for the families and unsound for the researcher just to ask them to "be natural for 10 minutes." Usually one or two specific tasks are chosen by the researcher so that all families start off with the same "set." Exactly what that task is depends on the construct that interests the researcher. For example:

- If the topic under study is how families express and react to expressions of emotion, or how they deal with conflict, one might ask them to discuss a topic of current concern, such as "their last family disagreement."
- If one is interested in decision-making processes within a family, one might ask family members to plan a family meal or a vacation.
- If support for growth and development in adolescence is the focus of the research, one might pose questions for discussion about which the adolescent and parents are likely to disagree, like "what the best curfew time would be."
- If the research question involves studying babies, toddlers, or young children and their families, one might ask them to "play together as you might if you found yourself at home with nothing to do."
- If one is interested in whether one or two people dominate the conversation in a family or are clearly leaders, one would describe the task in an unstructured way so that participation was clearly optional ("you should talk about movies you've liked"), whereas if one wanted a sample of interaction behavior from every person in the family, one might structure the task so that every person had to take a turn ("everyone should go around the circle and say what their favorite movie is and why").

- If one is interested in subtle interaction patterns that are likely to be present in most types of conversation, having the family participate in a specific laboratory task makes more sense than if one is interested in rare but highly salient patterns, such as family blowups or reactions to broken household rules. In the latter case, researchers have sometimes chosen to collect data about naturally occurring incidents at home rather than in a laboratory.

These are just a few examples of how the topic of interest should influence the choice of task for families. Markman and Notarius (1987) have recommended that, in order to begin to establish some comparability across studies, all family researchers should begin to include at least one identical task (they recommend a real-life problem-solving discussion). While this cooperation and agreement among researchers would certainly be useful (and unprecedented!), it is also important to make sure that a task is selected in each study that will allow the construct of interest to emerge. Box 4.1 includes a brief description of a few commonly used family observation tasks, with references to studies that have reported data from those tasks.

MINIMIZING THE ARTIFICIALITY
OF THE OBSERVATION

It is undeniable that these types of observed family interactions are somewhat artificial. Since is unethical to observe or videotape people in a research study without their prior knowledge, however, one always faces the possibility that families' interactions are, in some important way, altered by this knowledge or by their wanting to appear a certain way for the researcher. A number of steps can be taken to reduce this problem. (Gilbert & Christensen [1985] have written a thoughtful discussion of the issue.) First, one can pick a topic or task that will be *interesting* to the family because the more engaged in the task they are, the more the family members will forget that they are being observed and the more realistic and typical their interactions will be. Next, one can provide an honest and believable rationale for the whole research study in general, and for the task specifically. If families can make sense of and accept the importance of a study, they are more likely to focus on the task at hand than on the artificiality of it. Also, to some extent one can minimize the artificiality of the whole observation by keeping the camera and microphone equipment and/or coders out of sight (even

---

BOX 4.1
Family Interaction Tasks and
Examples of Studies in Which They Were Used

1. *Plan Something Together.* Families are asked to plan some activity together (for example, a family meal or a 2-week vacation) while being observed. Often some basic guidelines are given ("you have an unlimited budget," or "specify where you'll be each day and what you'll do there"), but the family members are given a fairly free hand to tackle the problem as they see fit. The system is often used when investigators are less interested in eliciting conflict and more interested in maximizing the participation of all members (see Grotevant and Cooper, 1985).

2. *Revealed Differences Task.* Each participating member of the family is first asked to complete some kind of questionnaire or interview, committing himself or herself to some position. Investigators have used questionnaires about such topics as family process, moral dilemma interviews, and lists of common curfews and rules to elicit initial responses. Then, the family members are united, and one or more items from the questionnaires on which family members initially disagreed are presented to the group. They are told that they did not all agree and are asked to come to some agreed-upon answer together. The task forces some degree of conflict into the family, and thus has been useful to investigators interested in such factors as conflict, dominance, and power (see Hauser et al., 1984).

3. *Unrevealed Differences Task.* This task is very similar in procedure and goal to the Revealed Differences Task, but the fact that there was disagreement at the individual level is "not revealed" to the family. They are left to discover this or not, as they will, during their discussion (see Ferreira 1963).

4. *Cognitive Problem-Solving.* The family is asked to perform a cognitive problem together, rather than engage in a discussion that would appear to be related to family process. An advantage of this approach is that families see the assignment as somewhat ambiguous and therefore are less likely or able to present themselves in a distorted way. Often, constructs can be coded that family members could not be expected to report about themselves. Families have been asked, for example, to put together color-form designs, build a tower of blocks, or sort cards into logical groupings (see Reiss 1981).

5. *Discussion of Typical Conflicts.* Here, families are asked to discuss a problem, issue, or conflict that is, in fact, real for them. Sometimes, they are given a long list of common problems from which to choose, and sometimes they generate the problem themselves. The assumption is that a realistic, meaningful problem to discuss will elicit realistic, meaningful interaction patterns from the family (see Doane et al., 1981).

6. *Stimulus Interpretation Tasks.* Families are given some type of ambiguous stimulus (such as a TAT card or a Rorschach card) to discuss or interpret together. The goal of studies using this task is usually to understand how family members communicate with each other (see Loveland, Wynne, & Singer, 1963).

(continued)

BOX 4.1
Continued

7. *SIMFAM*. Families are asked to play a game of some sort (e.g., video game, pinball, beanbag throwing) in which the rules are ambiguous and unknown to them. The family's task is to determine the rules of the game from feedback given during the game. The task was designed to measure such constructs as power, support, communication style, creativity, and problem-solving ability (see Straus and Tallman, 1971).

8. *Naturalistic, In-Home Observations*. Some researchers have chosen to observe families in their own homes as they go about their daily business of living, eating, cooking, and, of course, interacting with each other. Sometimes some guidelines or rules are set up (e.g., everyone in the family has to be in the home, they cannot sit and watch TV), but the goal is to capture a relatively unstructured, hence presumably more realistic, family interaction (see Patterson, 1984).

though the family knows they are there, not seeing them helps), and setting up the laboratory, if used, to resemble a living room.

Finally, one can try to assess the magnitude of reactivity present in a particular study (Haynes & Horn, 1982). At the conclusion of the observation, one can simply ask the family members how typical the observed sequence was of what happens at home. If it seems the family agrees that it was highly unusual ("we *never* get along that well," or "that's the first time my father hasn't told my mother what to do in years"), the data from those particular families could be analyzed with this information in mind. Haynes and Horn (1982) also discuss how changes in behavior rate over time (slope), statistical variability in the data, and discrepancies among presumably similar measures may be indicators of reactivity.

CHOOSING WHAT TO CODE

Think for a moment about what it would be like to have a 10- to 20-minute segment of a family interaction on videotape. Where would you start to describe the family? On what would you base your generalizations? Something one person said? The "sense" you get from the family? Some repeated pattern you observed? What if you have such a segment from 50 different families? What might seem important in one family might be totally absent in another. Perhaps the most critical task in designing an observational study of families is choosing the best focus and level of the coding to suit the needs of the research question. Choosing what to code in a family sequence can be compared to choosing how to describe a popular song. One can describe the lyrics, the tune, and/or the sentiment with which it is sung. Obviously these often overlap (you find few songs about unrequited love using a snappy major-key melody, sung with a lilt and a smile!), yet each component provides useful information about the song that is not tapped by the other components. One sad melody, for example, might be about un-requited love, a separation, or a loss. Capturing family sequences also depends on tapping these various interwoven levels. Gilbert and Christensen (1985) suggest that most family coding systems include measures from one or more of the following categories:

1. *Interpersonal Process (the "tune").* How do family members interact with each other, regardless of what they are saying? Does one person talk a lot while someone else hardly says anything at all? Is one person often interrupted? How much time follows each person's remarks before the next speaker begins? Does there seem to be an unwritten rule about the order of speaking (e.g., "whenever Tommy says something, Mom usually speaks next")? Is there a lot of tension in the family? Notice that in each of these cases, *what* is actually said is not considered at all. The emphasis here is on timing, sequencing, and proportion of the conversation dominated by particular members.

2. *Content of Verbalizations (the "lyrics").* Here, *what* is said is primary. Is what most of what one person says negative and pessimistic? Does one person usually get support and nurturance from other family members? Does one person ask all the questions? Are there pairs of family members that never seem to disagree with each other? Notice that these variables can be studied almost regardless of the task assigned to the family. Other content variables might be used that are specific to one particular task. For example, if the family was to plan a vacation together, one might code who made suggestions, who supported or disagreed with them, or whose idea was finally adopted.

3. *Affective Display (the "sentiment").* Nonverbal aspects of a family's inter-action are captured here. Is one person particularly sullen even when, on the content level, he seems to be cooperating? Are there "dirty looks," strained tones of voice, or hand gestures that suggest conflict between two people? Does one person appear to be particularly attentive, leaning forward, nodding, or smiling, even though she does not say anything? These variables would not be coded in either of the first two categories,

yet clearly are relevant. You have surely heard the same song sung by a few different people—the tune is the same, the lyrics are the same, but how they sing it, the amount of affect, the speed, and the backup instrumentation all differ, and the result can be quite different. These affective display variables are all comparable to "how the song is sung."

HOW TO CAPTURE WHAT IS
GOING ON: CODING VERSUS RATING

Within each of the above categories, one can code family interaction at a very specific, microlevel, or rate interaction at a more global, clinical, macrolevel. *Specific codes* tend to focus on smaller, more discrete units of behavior that, while sometimes more superficial, are easier to code reliably and easier to describe to the scientific community. Examples include "number of interruptions" or "proportion of total conversation exchanges made by each family member" (interpersonal process level), "number of disagreements" or "number of praises" (content level), and "proportion of remarks accompanied by a smile" or a minute-to-minute rating of each member's "involvement in the conversation" (affective level). A number of widely used code systems of this sort are described at the end of this chapter.

Note that at each level, there are several options concerning how to quantify the construct of interest. One can actually *count* a behavior or a sequence within some previously defined category, *time* the duration of a particular behavior, or *rate* the construct on some kind of scale. For example, if one is interested in the construct of marital discord, one could *count* the number of times each spouse makes a hostile, sarcastic, or insulting remark to the other; *time* the length of neutral or positive passages in the couples' conversations; or *rate* each 5-minute segment on a 7-point scale of compatibility. Obviously, the results of these methods would not be identical, and it is up to the researcher to choose the method that can most reliably and validly capture the phenomenon of interest.

Another way in which observational systems differ is in whether they are designed to include a record of every occurrence in the interaction period or, instead, to include a sampling of the behavior of the family during the observation. In some code systems, every event that occurs is recorded into one and only one category (e.g., mother asks question, then child asks different question, then mother answers child's question, then father answers mother's question, then father makes suggestion, then child says no, etc.). This procedure of continuously recording events has the benefit of including all that goes on in the family (at least as reflected in the categories used) during that interaction, of capturing both common and rare events, and of being useful in sequential analysis (see Chapter 6).

In other systems, an arbitrary time interval is chosen (like 10 seconds or 1 minute), and each person's behavior (e.g., the behavior going on at the moment the interval is over) is coded once during that interval. This interval-recording procedure is most useful when the behavior of interest is not very rare (because rare events might not have occurred just at the moment the coding is to take place, and therefore would be lost), and when the interval can be short enough that important events are not lost; it has the advantage of efficiency and the disadvantage of inaccuracy.

Still other systems present the observer with an arbitrary signal to record what behavior is occurring at that moment (e.g., every 5 minutes, or at a randomly presented tone). A number of excellent articles and books have been written about these and other types of observational methods, their advantages and disadvantages, and the appropriate methods of determining their validity and interjudge reliability (see the "Recommended Reading" section at the end of this chapter). Since many of the principles are the same whether one is observing families, individuals, or pigeons, the principles will not be reviewed here.

In contrast to these microlevel codes, *global ratings* tend to focus on whole interaction sessions or the overall sense of a larger segment of interaction. While sometimes requiring many hours of intensive or clinical training, they can capture in a few variables much of the complexity of family interaction. Examples include overall ratings, perhaps based on the entire 10- to 20-minute observation, of one person's assertiveness in the family; of who seems to have the power to influence the family; of the whole family's task-orientedness; of dyadic conflict; or of enmeshment, alliances, or any number of clinical concepts of theoretical importance. Carlson and Grotevant (1987a) provide a very useful review of observational rating scales and a description of their strengths and limitations. An interesting exchange in response to their article, with special emphasis on comparing the utility of coding versus rating scales for capturing family process, is provided by Cowan (1987), Coyne (1987), Fisher (1987), and Carlson and Grotevant (1987b).

SAMPLE FAMILY OBSERVATIONAL SYSTEMS

While many researchers choose to develop their own observation systems so that the specific focus of their research question is addressed, there is certainly a lot to be said for researchers using systems already in the literature. Only in this way can we start to develop a data base in which results from various studies can be compared. Using a published system saves each researcher the enormous task of developing and standardizing a new system, and keeps the literature relatively free of studies with small sample sizes and limited psychometric support. The more researchers use the same systems, the more valuable information about their validity and reliability accrues, making them, in turn, even more useful for future research. Thus if your research question can be adequately addressed by an existing, widely used tool, we encourage you to use it instead of making up your own. An example of coding a family discussion is found in Box 4.2.

Several of the existing widely used tools one can use are described below. As with the self-report measures described in Chapter 3, this list is not meant to be exhaustive; rather, the list is representative of the kinds of constructs and methods other family researchers have used. Note that the systems represent a wide range of theoretical perspectives: developmental, psychoanalytic, social learning, systemic. We list systems first that deal with marital/couple dyads, then parent-child dyads, and then those that deal with families, including parents and at least one child. We include a parent-child dyad assessment tool because some questions still warrant a dyadic approach, but the reader is reminded that the interaction between a parent-child dyad must never be assumed to be a proxy for a family interaction that includes both parents. The family observation systems are further divided into those primarily derived to distinguish problem from nonproblem families and those derived to capture the family as a context for development, a classification suggested by Grotevant and Carlson (1987). (Also see Jacob [1975, 1987] and Doane [1978] for a discussion of observed differences between problem and nonproblem families.) In some cases, the designation to one of these two categories was a bit arbitrary; in fact, many family researchers are concerned about describing normal family process *and* are interested in whether the dimensions they observe distinguish problem from nonproblem families. Several articles that review the methodology of these systems and that were useful in compiling the following summaries are listed at the end of this chapter; much more

---

BOX 4.2
A Sample of Coding a Family Discussion

In the course of a study of family alliances, Copeland (1990) asked families to be videotaped while discussing, among other things, what they would plan for a special dinner were they to have an unlimited budget. She coded the discussions using a modification of the Family Alliances Coding System, or FACS, by Gilbert et al. (1981). In this system, each speaking event is coded for (a) who spoke, (b) to whom the utterance was directed, (c) the content of the utterance, (d) the affect accompanying the utterance, and, where relevant, (e) about or for whom the speaker was speaking. Some of the content codes in the code system are:

1. *Structure* (ST). Statement designed to facilitate the responding of another
2. *Personal Statement* (PS). Neutral statement without implications for alliances
3. *Guiding Question* (GQ). Question designed to express benign lack of support with suggestion made previously by encouraging person to reconsider his or her position
4. *Agree-Approve* (AA). Statement indicating that the speaker favors a specific statement or suggestion of another
5. *Positive Coalition* (PC). Statement indicating two people will engage or have engaged in a pleasing activity together
6. *Positive Appeal* (PA). Comments designed to elicit support for self

A small segment of a discussion by two parents and their 10- and 8-year-old daughters (called Child 1 and 2, respectively) follows, with some of the coding noted to the right.

	To Whom	Content	Affect
Child 1: OK, well, so what are we going to have?	all	ST	+
Child 2: I dunno.	C1	PS	0
Father: Shall we have a theme or just pick out foods we like?	C1+2	ST	0
Mother: Do you have a favorite thing in the whole world?	C1+2	ST	0
Child 1: How about, well, one of the courses that I think would be great; well, I love fettucine.	Mo	PS	+
Mother: And you want a whole course of fettucine?	C1	GQ	0
Child 1: Yeah.	Mo	PS	0
Child 2: Yeah!	Mo	AA	+

(continued)

Box 4.2
Continued

	To Whom	Content	Affect
Mother: Well, do you want plain fettucine or, like, alfredo, with the cream on it?	C1+2	ST	0
Child 2: Alfredo.	Mo	PS	0
Father: Mom and I had that last week at the Johnsons and it was really great.	C1+2	PC	+
Child 2: And let's have a salad.	all	PS	0
Mother: We could have a salad, but I'd like to think about the main course before I decide on things that go with it.	C2	ST	0
Child 2: I want just, like, a small little salad, don't you?	C1	PA	0
Child 1: Yeah.	C2	PS	0
Mother: Um-hm.	C2	PS	0
Child 2: Just a regular basic salad, OK?	Mo	PA	0
Mother: Well, but if we could have anything we want, there are some wonderful, special things we could put in the salad.	C2	ST	0

Note that the affect ratings are not always discernable from a transcript; the segment was coded while watching the videotape. For example, when the older girl said the first sentence, she had a big smile on her face and was bouncing up and down on her chair; hence the positive affect rating.

detail about the systems, what they really measure and how, and their strengths and weaknesses are given in these reviews, and the reader is strongly urged to consult them.

Marital/Couple Observation Systems

Marital Interaction Coding System, or MICS. This system (original version by Hops, Wills, Patterson, & Weiss [1972]; a more recent revision, MICS-III, by Weiss & Summers [1983]) is important both because it has been used so often and because it has spawned many other code systems. The MICS' emphasis is on describing marital interaction, especially when the couple is dealing with conflict, and is based on a behavioral or social learning framework that focuses on the specific behavior each partner brings to an interaction. The participating couple is asked to discuss, for 10 minutes, an issue or problem either that is relevant to them or that was chosen from a list of topics designed to generate conflict; discussions are audiotaped or videotaped and coded later.

The MICS-III includes 32 behavioral codes of things either member of the couple can do or say. These have been combined into eight dimensions: problem description, blame (e.g., complain, criticize), make positive or negative proposal for change (or compromise), validation (e.g., agree, approve), invalidation (e.g., interrupt, deny responsibility), facilitation (e.g., paraphrase), nonverbal affect (e.g., smile, positive physical contact), and irrelevant (e.g., comments about the study). Two coders record what each partner says or does in a sequential fashion (making it suitable for sequential analysis; see Chapter 6), in 30-second blocks.

The focus of reliability assessment for the MICS-III has been mostly on interobserver agreement and generally has been maintained above the 70% level; since two coders always code each tape, disagreements can be resolved by discussion. The measure successfully has distinguished between distressed and nondistressed couples (Birchler, Weiss, & Vincent, 1975) and between those who have and have not seen benefits from marital therapy (Jacobson, 1977). In some cases, it also has been found to be related to self-report measures of marital satisfaction (Haynes, Follingstad, & Sullivan, 1979). Gottman and Krokoff (1989) used the MICS to demonstrate that some aspects of marital interaction (e.g., conflict engagement) could be "dysfunctional" concurrently yet predict improvement in marital satisfaction 3 years later. Other aspects (e.g., wife's positive verbal behavior) were related to concurrent marital satisfaction and to deterioration in satisfaction after 3 years. Strengths of the code system are that it has been revised through the years in response to new empirical and methodological developments in the field, and that it has been used often by researchers with a wide variety of questions. A weakness is that its construct validity has not been investigated thoroughly (Filsinger, 1983; Markman & Notarius, 1987), although this becomes less true the more the MICS-III continues to be used in published studies.

Couples Interaction Scoring System (CISS—pronounced "kiss" not "sis"—it is a couple code, after all). The MICS and the CISS (Gottman, Markman, & Notarius, 1977) are similar in a number of ways, and have influenced and been influenced by each other over time (in fact, see Gottman & Krokoff, 1989, for an example of a study using both measures). Although the CISS shares the goal of capturing the process of interaction of distressed and nondistressed couples as they engage in problem-solving conversations, the CISS differs importantly from the MICS in including a content *and* a nonverbal code for every unit of behavior by the speaker and a nonverbal code for the listener in every coded unit. In the MICS, nonverbal behavior may or may not be coded at a given moment. In the CISS procedure, couples are asked to discuss for 10 to 15 minutes a problem they are having, a problem not directly relevant to the couple but which is often conflict producing, or, in other studies, how their day went. Each unit of speech is coded into one of 28 content codes which, as with the MICS, are usually collapsed into eight dimensions: problem talk, mind reading, proposing solution, communication talk, agreement, disagreement, summarizing talk, and summarizing self. Nonverbal codes of the speaker and listener are judged by a different coder on the basis of a scan of the person's facial expression (e.g., smile, frown, head nod, sneer), voice tone (e.g., caring, cold, tense, warm) and body position (e.g., touching, open arms, rude gestures, hand tension); a summary judgment of positive, negative, or neutral is made for each unit. If interobserver agreement falls below 80%, tapes are recoded. Cohen's kappa for content and nonverbal codes has been found to exceed .71 (Gottman, 1979). The concurrent validity of the measure has been supported by findings that distressed and nondistressed couples score differently, especially on the nonverbal codes and in analyses of the sequences of their behavior. Distressed couples, not surprisingly, were found to be more negative in affect, and to continue negative interactions longer than nondistressed couples who were able to avoid a "cross-complaining" mode ("Oh, yeah, well if that's what you think, I'll tell you something else I don't like . . ."; see Gottman [1979]; Gottman et al. [1977]). While the strengths of including nonverbal coding and the possibility of sequential analysis have been made clear by these validity studies, the code system will profit from more attention to its predictive and construct validity (Filsinger, 1983; Markman & Notarius, 1987).

Parent-Child Interaction Observation Systems

Response-Class Matrix. The Response-Class Matrix (Mash, Terdal, & Anderson, 1973), a system of capturing the interplay of parents' and children's behavior as they interact with each other, was developed before sequential analysis techniques were widely used. It is based in a behavioral framework emphasizing the role of one person's behavior as both a consequent of the prior behavior of another person, and as an antecedent to that other person's subsequent behavior. It was designed originally to code the behavior of mothers interacting with their handicapped children, but has also captured important interaction processes of hyperactive children and their mothers, of siblings where one is hyperactive and the other is not, and of divorcing mothers and their children (see Mash & Barkley, 1986, for a review).

Most often in uses of the Response-Class Matrix, dyads are videotaped while doing a structured task (e.g., putting toys away, building a tower blindfolded) and an unstructured task (e.g., free play, making a crafts project), in a simulation of at-home behavior, for 10 to 15 minutes each. Two coders code each tape using a time-sampling approach. Every 15 seconds, one codes the child's response to the mother's most recent behavior (e.g., child complies with mother's command), and the other codes the mother's behavior as a response to the child's most recent behavior (mother gives a command after child disobeys).

While categories have differed slightly across studies, most include similar categories of behavior for mother and children: command, command-question ("Don't you want to try this one?"), comply, noncomply, praise, question, negative, interaction (neutral statement or play), and no interaction (ignoring or non sequitur remarks). Thus individual behavior categories for each dyad member can be tallied (e.g., "total number of commands given, regardless of how other person responded"), as can particular antecedent-consequent sequences (e.g., "total number of mother commands with which the child complied"). The system has been used to describe synchrony in and quality of interaction, maternal directiveness, child compliance, and related constructs. Interobserver agreement is maintained at above the 80% level, and concurrent validity of the code system is attested to by its ability to differentiate dyads that include problem children (e.g., handicapped, hyperactive, behavior disordered) versus nonproblem children (Mash & Barkley, 1986). This system is best seen as a compromise between the advantages of efficiency and lower labor-intensity of a time-sampling procedure and the benefits of a system that allows for sequential analysis.

**Family Interaction Observation Systems Designed
to Assess Differences Between Distressed and Nondistressed Families**

Interaction Code. This system (Mishler & Waxler, 1968), included here mostly because it has had such a heuristic impact on the field of family observation, was developed to try to capture differences (hypothesized to be etiological ones) between families that included a schizophrenic child versus families that did not. In Mishler and Waxler's study, a schizophrenic child with his or her two parents (in the clinical families) were asked to complete the Revealed Differences Task (see Box 4.1). Discussions were audiotaped; transcriptions were coded sentence by sentence in the following ways: who spoke to whom, stimulus (e.g., command, question, acknowledgment), response (e.g., complete versus partial acknowledgment), affect, focus (e.g., agree, disagree, own opinion, item content), evidence of tension (repetition, incomplete phrase), interruptions, metacommunication (statements about the communication process), and instrumental-expressive questions and answers (derived from Bales, 1950).

These codes were used by Mishler and Waxler (1968) to try to portray family members' expressiveness, power, speech disruption, responsiveness, and strategies for attention and control. In this study, interobserver agreement stayed above 85%, and the validity of the system was supported by the finding that several clusters of codes did, in fact, discriminate families with and without schizophrenic children. This early study was important in demonstrating that both content (e.g., support and validation) and process codes (e.g., interruptions and talk time) can be reliably coded and related to important clinical dimensions. Even though later code systems have improved the assessment of dominance, the nonverbal aspects of affect, and speech disturbance, many family observers acknowledge their debt to Mishler and Waxler for this early work (Grotevant & Carlson, 1987; Markman & Notarius, 1987).

Family Interaction Coding System (FICS). This measure (Patterson, Ray, Shaw, & Cobb, 1969; Reid, 1978) is based on a social learning analysis of coercion and social aggression within families. The authors' work began with the study of aggressive children and the assumption that their families provided a crucial environment for the maintenance of aggression. It is a widely used tool in studies of conduct-disordered children and has spawned a number of other related observational systems (e.g., another parent-child dyad tool, the Dyadic Parent-Child Interaction Coding System; Robinson & Eyberg, 1981). Families typically are observed in their homes, but in a semistructured setting; that is, some rules are established to maintain some degree of comparability and utility of the data (e.g., all family members must be present, they cannot be watching TV).

In the FICS procedure, families are coded live, with the advantage of needing no obtrusive equipment, but with the disadvantage of having a researcher in the living room and of not being able to replay scenes during coding. One person is randomly chosen to be the target of observation for 5 minutes, after which time another family member is chosen; various family members are watched in 5-minute segments, for a minimum total of 70 minutes. The behavior of each target is coded, and then the reactions to that behavior by others is coded. The data obtained can thus be analyzed with sequential techniques (see Chapter 6).

There are currently 29 codes in the FICS: 14 aversive ones (e.g., cry, disapprove, humiliate, tease) and 15 prosocial ones (e.g., approval, compliance, laugh, play). Interobserver agreement has been found to be sufficiently high, and the FICS has been found to be generalizable across observers, settings, and targets. The validity of the system is supported by studies that show the FICS to differentiate between families with normal and antisocial children (see Patterson, 1982, for a review) and, even more compellingly, by studies that show it can differentiate between families with socially aggressive children and families with hyperactive children or children who steal (Grotevant & Carlson, 1987). Thus the FICS seems to be an excellent measure for studying families with conduct-disordered children, especially because it is so widely used. It is, naturally, less useful for more general or for other specific research questions. Indeed, Patterson (1982) himself notes that despite the inclusion of 15 prosocial codes, the code system is more sensitive to aversive than positive interactions.

Affective Style Measure. Working with high-risk adolescents within a framework emphasizing degree of expressed emotion within families, Doane, Goldstein, and Rodenick (1981) developed this family observation coding system to try to predict which adolescents would develop psychiatric disorders and, of those, what the likely course of the disorder and treatment would be. Families are asked to complete Revealed Differences Tasks or to discuss a relevant family problem, once with the adolescent alone with each parent and once as a triad. The parents' style in interacting with their adolescents is coded with an event-sampling procedure for criticisms (which can be either "personal"—harsh ones directed to the child—or "benign"—circumscribed or matter-of-fact), guilt induction (implications that the child is at fault and that the parent is upset), intrusiveness (implications that the parents can read the children's thoughts, feelings, or motivations), and support (positive supportive statements). Adequate interobserver agreement (Cohen's kappa over .78) has been reported. The measure has successfully predicted psychiatric status (Doane et al., 1981) and, in combination with Singer and Wynne's (1966) Communication Deviance Index, has predicted schizophrenia in young adulthood. Clearly, this is a promising and valuable tool, though the narrow focus of the codes makes its utility somewhat limited.

The Home Observation Assessment Method (HOAM). An observation tool that is quite different from all the others described in this section, the HOAM (Steinglass, 1976) focuses on in-home naturalistic movement and interaction patterns. While potentially useful for nondistressed families, it has mostly been used to study families with an alcoholic member. Observers enter the home for several hours and code which rooms people are in, the physical distance between people when they talk with each other, how much they actually interact with each other and what they say (e.g., task orientation, problem solving, information exchange), the affective level of their interactions, and the outcome of the interactions. From these measures, researchers can derive estimates of such constructs as distance regulation, stability versus variability, or level of engagement. Kappa coefficients have suggested that adequate interobserver agreement is possible, and the measure has successfully discriminated alcoholic from nonalcoholic families (Steinglass, 1979) and has predicted the course of alcoholism over time (Steinglass, Tislenko, & Reiss, 1985). Note that in contrast to most other family observation tools, this measure takes place in the home, no specific task is assigned to the family, and the emphasis is not exclusively on verbal exchange.

Beavers-Timberlawn Scales. Two rating scales based on the Beavers Systems Model of Family Functioning (see Chapter 2) have been reported (Beavers, 1982; Lewis, Beavers, Gossett, & Phillips, 1976). The Beavers-Timberlawn Family Evaluation Scale is a 14-item measure consisting of 6 major scales: Family Structure, Mythology, Goal-Directed Negotiation, Autonomy, Family Affect, and Global Health/Pathology. Each item is rated on a 5-point scale. The Beavers-Timberlawn Centripetal/Centrifugal Family Style Scale is a 7-item measure in which various aspects of family interaction (e.g., social presentation, positive expression of feelings) are rated on a 5-point scale from "centrifugal" to "centripetal." Both rating scales have the advantage of being grounded in theory, but both suffer from having some scales with inadequate reliability (although experienced family therapists seem to be more reliable) and limited evidence of validity.

Family Interaction Observation Systems Designed to Assess the Family as a Context for Development

Family Discourse Code. The Family Discourse Code (Condon, Cooper, & Grotevant, 1984; Grotevant & Cooper, 1985) was designed to tap those aspects of families that facilitate or inhibit adolescents' familial individuation and connectedness. It represents a creative integration of several different theoretical underpinnings, including family systems and developmental theories about individuation, and on research on communication processes. Families are asked to plan something together; observations are made and audiotaped at home.

Asserting that conversational bids should be thought of as having two functions—to respond to previous utterances (i.e., even a change of topic indicates some kind of response) and to further the discourse—these researchers code each utterance into one of several "response" categories (e.g., agrees, answers request, complies) *and* into one of several "move" categories (e.g., suggests action, requests information). The various codes thus reflect the family and adolescents' self-assertion, permeability, and validation which, in turn, have been shown to reflect the degree of individuation and connectedness in the family. These constructs, in turn, have been shown to be related to adolescents' identity exploration (Grotevant & Cooper, 1985).

Family Constraining and Enabling Coding System (CECS). Like the Family Discourse Code, the CECS (Hauser, Powers, Weiss, Follansbee, & Bernstein, 1983) also focuses on those aspects of families that facilitate (or enable) the psychological development of adolescents. The theoretical framework of the CECS, however, is more psychoanalytic, and emphasizes how parents affect adolescents' development

(Steirlin, 1974). Families complete a Revealed Differences Task (focusing on several moral dilemma questions, a task likely to have special interest to adolescents) while being audiotaped. Using an event-sampling procedure, "key events" (where the adolescent takes a stand about an issue) are coded from audio transcriptions as to how they are handled within the family. Parents' reactions to the adolescent are coded as being cognitively constraining (e.g., withholding, judgmental), cognitively enabling (e.g., problem solving, curiosity), affectively constraining (e.g., devaluing), or affectively enabling (e.g., acceptance). In addition, the adolescent's response to the parent is then coded as constraining or enabling, as is the progression of discourse (e.g., change of topic, increase or decrease of participation). Acceptable levels of kappa agreement have been reported. As predicted, both parental adolescent enabling and constraining have been shown to be related to adolescents' level of ego development as measured on Loevinger's (1976) ego development scale (Hauser et al., 1984).

Interaction Process Coding System (IPCS). The IPCS (Bell, Bell, & Cornwell, 1982) is yet another coding system designed to assess the interactional processes between adolescents and their parents in nonclinical families, and the relationships of these processes to the adolescents' ego development. Based on family systems, communications, and developmental theories, the system is used to code audiotapes of families engaging (in their homes) in a Revealed Differences Task. Unlike many other systems that prohibit the presence of more than two parents and one child, this system allows for the participation of up to five people (including either one or two parents) at a time. The speaker and recipient (i.e., who was addressed) of each speech unit are coded, as are the topic of each unit of speech (e.g., whether it is about the task or not), the focus of the speech (e.g., behavior, feelings, ideas), amount of support inherent in the speech (on a 7-point scale), and level of validation of the other. From these codes, the investigators have been able to study the cognitive validation, affective support, and level and type of power present in the family interaction. Little reliability and validity data are available, though interobserver agreement has been reported to exceed 71%. The system holds promise because of the possibility of including single parents and more than one child; more data on the validity of the system with these larger family groups are needed.

Global Family Interaction Scales (FIS-II). The FIS-II (Riskin, 1982) is a rating scale that extends the information obtained with the original FIS (Riskin & Faunce, 1972), a coding measure. The FIS-II involves rating families on 17 dimensions of family process (e.g., humor, agreement, intensity, intrusiveness). The measure has not been used extensively in research, so evidence for its reliability and validity is scant, though promising.

SUMMARY OF OBSERVATIONAL SYSTEMS

Note that by and large, the modal family-level system reviewed here centers on the study of two parents and one adolescent, discussing a topic assigned by the researcher, in a laboratory. The literature that has grown from these studies has certainly augmented our understanding of adolescents and their mental health in an unprecedented way. However, it would be useful if investigators would begin to explore family interaction in new directions. We need to be able to study different family forms (single parents, more than one child at a time, more than two generations) and families in which the children cannot be expected to engage in a long verbal (codable!) interchange (as with young children). The trade-offs between the methodological control available in laboratories and the realism of in-home studies needs to be continually assessed. And the impact of various family tasks on the kinds of data produced by families also needs to be explored further. Notice that some of the systems reviewed here attempt to capture family process in some global way thought to represent core dimensions of the family, while others have openly focused on quite specific aspects of family interchange. This diversity is probably a good thing, as family theory does not yet have definitive answers as to what makes the most functional and healthful family process.

EXERCISES

1. Send two of your friends out of the room temporarily. Plan a very simple task for them to do when they return; for example, you might plan for one to play the role of a child and the other to play a parent, and ask them to draw a picture together on the blackboard. Decide beforehand on several

aspects of the interaction to code; try your hand at coding something you can count (e.g., the number of suggestions the "parent" makes about what to draw), something you can time (e.g., the number of seconds the "child" is actually drawing on the blackboard), and something you can rate (e.g., how much fun the "parent-child" dyad seemed to have). After observing for a few minutes, decide on five to six categories of behavior that seem to capture most of the interaction (e.g., parent makes suggestion, parent praises, parent criticizes, parent asks question, child complies, child draws). Assign each category an abbreviation (e.g., parent makes suggestion = PMS), and then try to record every event in sequence as the dyad interacts again. Finally, try an interval recording scheme (e.g., have your instructor announce 15-second intervals; at each announcement, record whether or not the pair is discussing the picture). Having tried each of these approaches, what unexpected difficulties did you have? How did you agree with your classmates? Did one type of system result in higher agreement among you than other types?

2. Say you were interested in each of the following research questions and wanted to include an observational component to your study of the issue. For each question, where would be the best place to conduct the observation and why; who should be present; what would you ask the families to do during the observation to best elicit the constructs of interest; what are 10 to 12 things you would most likely want to code; and what would be the best coding approach to take? Because all decisions of these types necessarily involve some kind of compromise, discuss what problems might occur or limitations ensue from each of your decisions.

    (a) Do families with terminally ill children interact differently with each other than families with healthy children?

    (b) Are there differences in how "democratic" families are with high- versus low-achieving children?

    (c) Do parents raise their children the way they themselves were raised?

RECOMMENDED READING

Bakeman, R., & Gottman, J. M. (1986). *Observing interaction: An introduction to sequential analysis.* Cambridge: Cambridge University Press. (See especially Chapters 1 through 5 for a discussion of basic observational methods.)

Carlson, C. I., & Grotevant, H. D. (1987). A comparative review of family rating scales: Guidelines for clinicians and researchers. *Journal of Family Psychology, 1,* 62-65.

Doane, J. A. (1978). Family interaction and communication deviance in disturbed and normal families. *Family Process, 17,* 357-373.

Filsinger, E. E. (1983). Choices among marital observation coding systems. *Family Process, 22,* 317-335.

Foster, S. L., & Cone, J. D. (1986). Design and use of direct observation procedures. In A. R. Ciminero, K. S. Calhoun, & H. E. Adams (Eds.), *Handbook of behavioral assessment* (2nd ed., pp. 253-324). New York: John Wiley.

Gilbert, R., & Christensen, A. (1985). Observational assessment of marital and family interaction: Methodological considerations. In L. L'Abate (Ed.), *The handbook of family psychology and therapy* (Vol. 2, pp. 961-987). Homewood, IL: Dorsey.

Grotevant, H. D., & Carlson, C. I. (1987). Family interaction coding systems: A descriptive review. *Family Process, 26,* 49-74.

Jacob, T. (1975). Family interaction in disturbed and normal families: A methodological and substantive review. *Psychological Bulletin, 82,* 33-65.

Jacob, T., & Tennenbaum, D. L. (1988). *Family assessment: Rationale, methods, and future directions.* New York: Plenum.

Markman, H. J., & Notarius, C. I. (1987). Coding marital and family interaction: Current status. In T. Jacob (Ed.), *Family interaction and psychopathology: Theories, methods, and findings* (pp.329-390). New York: Plenum.

5

Taking Advantage of Existing Data Sources

In the preceding chapters, we have discussed studies that are complex in design and/or conception, and that may have been difficult, expensive, and/or time consuming to conduct. The mere task of scheduling a family's participation in a research study (juggling the work and school schedules of the family and the research team and *their* families, the children's after-school activities, illnesses, and other considerations) sets the stage for the complexity that may follow. One may then be faced with a working model that demands the collection of measures of a relatively large number of constructs from a variety of informants, assumptions about how family process manifests itself that require highly trained coders to interpret observational or interview data, and/ or design demands that require repeated assessments of families. Thus the conduct of this kind of family research study is rarely taken on lightly, and the progress of the field of family research is necessarily slowed.

Some investigators have turned, creatively, to existing data sources to address some of these concerns, and to explore new and different research questions. By using data sets from already completed studies on related topics, from public records, various family and social archives, and large-scale surveys, family researchers have been able to extend their investigations in new and important ways. (See Stewart, 1984, for an extended discussion of secondary analysis.)

SECONDARY ANALYSIS OF DATA

Secondary analysis involves using existing data sets to ask questions not asked by the original researcher, or to ask the same questions in new ways. We use this term broadly, to include analysis of data sets designed for other purposes *and* of data sets, such as large-scale surveys or census records, that may have been collected specifically for the use of both current and unspecified future purposes. Many research studies involve the collection of very rich and/or extensive data that cannot be analyzed thoroughly by a single researcher or within a single theoretical framework. Interviews, written narratives, observations, questionnaires, and demographic surveys can usually be read with new perspectives and new insights on identical or related topics; this is called secondary analysis.

There are three general types of existing data that are most commonly used in secondary analysis of family issues. One is the sets of raw and/or coded interview, questionnaire, psychological test, and/or observational measures collected for one purpose that can be reanalyzed or used in follow-up studies to address new questions about families. For example, Elder, Nguyen, and Caspi (1985) used data from the Oakland Growth Study, a longitudinal study of 167 Californian children born in 1920 and 1921, to address questions about how economic hardship, parenting, and children's behavior are related, questions that were not part of the original study. Parenting behavior was coded, retroactively, from available interviews with mothers and observations of parents. Information about the children was quantified on the basis of a Q-sort measure. Other kinds of measures used in the analyses were chosen from the many available measures on the families (e.g., ratings of children's attractiveness made at the time of original data collection). The authors used findings from these new and original scores to suggest economic hardship adversely affected the psychosocial well-being of girls, especially less attractive girls, but did not affect boys.

Data of this type might be obtained directly from the original researcher or through a data archive center. The Henry A. Murray Center at Radcliffe College, for example, houses the original or computer-accessible data of over 190 investigations that concern the study of lives, human development, and social change, especially investigations focused on women's lives and issues of concern to women. These issues include women's work and career, education, mental health, widowhood, and, of most importance here, family life. The Murray Center holds such raw data sets as:

- *Sears, Maccoby, and Levin's "Patterns of Childrearing Study."* Transcribed interviews and computer-accessible data from a study in the early 1950s of 379 suburban mothers of kindergarten children about their childrearing practices and values; includes several follow-up assessments.
- *Grossman's "Pregnancy and Parenthood Project."* Audiotapes and raw and computer-accessible data from rating and self-report scales from a

6-year longitudinal study of 100 couples expecting a baby, with follow-up into early childhood, conducted in the 1970s to the 1980s.
- *Belle's "Stress and Families Project."* Raw data, including child observations and parent interviews, and computer-accessible data from a 1981 study of the relationship between life situation and mental health in 43 low-income mothers, fathers, and children.
- *Bozett's "Children of Gay Fathers Study."* Interview transcripts from 19 children (ages 14 to 35) of gay fathers, focusing on communication about homosexuality and the current relationship between father and child.

In some cases, raw data are not available, but access to the data, as coded by the original researcher (e.g., interview responses, observational measures, questionnaire responses, psychological test scores), is. While having access only to the codes rather than the original product obviously does not allow new types of coding by the secondary analyst, new questions can be asked by grouping subjects in a new way, relating new groups of variables to each other based on new questions, and/or using the data for follow-up or replication purposes. For example, the Murray Center holds computer access to the coded tests and questionnaires from subsets of two longitudinal studies—the Berkeley Guidance Study, begun with families of 21-month-old children in 1929, and the Oakland Growth Study, described earlier (see Jones, Bayley, Macfarlane, & Honzik, 1971, and Elder, 1974, respectively, for descriptions of studies based on these two data sets).

Murray Center resources are available to undergraduate and graduate students, faculty, and researchers. Computer tapes can be made available to local universities, but raw data must be analyzed at the Center (10 Garden Street, Cambridge, MA 02138). Having access to existing raw and coded data provides many exciting opportunities for researchers.

Alternatively, family researchers have turned to survey research for help in answering their questions. Some survey data sets include responses that directly concern family issues; others include items from which family-related variables can be derived. For example, Jackson's National Survey of Black Americans, conducted in 1979-1980, sampled 2,107 black adult U.S. citizens (Jackson, Tucker, & Bowman, 1982). Survey questions tapped such areas as neighborhood-community integration, crime and community contact, the role of religion and the church, physical and mental health, self-esteem, and interaction with family and friends. The National Longitudinal Survey of Labor Market Experience 1966-1986 included five cohorts of men and women, interviewed at least every 2 years on issues of labor market behavior and experience, education and training, and, for the youth cohort, issues of fertility, pre- and postnatal care, child care, and alcohol and drug use. (Nonsurvey data are also available from the 5,000 children of the female youth cohort assessed in 1986, including home observations, temperament and developmental measures, and family history.)

The Murray Center holds many survey research data sets on computer tape. In addition, an excellent source of social science data, including large survey data sets, is the Inter-university Consortium for Political and Social Research (ICPSR) at the University of Michigan. Over 325 colleges and universities in 14 countries belong to this consortium and thus have access to machine-readable data tapes of studies on individual attitudes and social experiences related to all social science disciplines. For example, there are archival holdings relating to historical and contemporary population characteristics, community and urban studies, conflict, aggression, violence, wars, health care, political behavior and attitudes, and social institutions and behavior. The 1988-1989 *Guide to Resources and Services* provides summaries of the archived studies, references to publications using the data sets, and procedures for using the archive.

A third source of existing data that has been fruitful for family researchers is data collected originally primarily for legal, medical, political, or other nonpsychosocial reasons. Webb, Campbell, Schwartz, and Sechrest (1966) discuss these data as "running records," ongoing, continuing records of a society that can be exploited by social scientists. Rank (1987), for instance, analyzed data in the computerized records of the Aid to Families with Dependent Children, Food Stamp, and Medicaid programs to examine the relationship between the probability of being married and such factors as race, having a young child in the home, and wife's employment status. Oster (1987) collected data on alimony awards from the public records of one particular courthouse on all divorces for which financial statements were available during a 6-month period. These records typically included information on size of award, lump-sum payments, and a narrative on other characteristics of the couple, so Oster was able to describe the role of family and relationship characteristics in affecting alimony determinations. Erez and Tontodonato (1989) examined the domestic incident reports filed in one year by 28 police departments in a single county in order to study rates of child-to-parent and parent-to-child abuse. Koo, Suchindran, and Griffith (1987) analyzed data from the 1980 Current Population

Survey of the Bureau of the Census and found that women who experienced marital disruption and remarriage (which is asked directly on the questionnaire) by age 45 took longer to finish their reproduction (which was coded from the dates of birth of the children) and that educated women took less time. Similar kinds of family-related questions might be approached through analysis of medical, school, or other such records. Besides using such records as the primary data source (as in the examples above), they may also be useful in providing background information about data sets of interest. For example, if a researcher is interested in reanalyzing data from a sample of single parent families collected in 1960, census reports from that year could be very useful in describing the sociocultural background (e.g., prevalence of single parents, divorce rates) at the time. The Interuniversity Consortium for Political and Social Research includes many such data sets, including the Current Population Surveys from the Bureau of the Census.

ADVANTAGES OF SECONDARY ANALYSIS

Colby (1982) has pointed out some of the advantages and disadvantages of secondary analysis, and the reader interested in this approach will find her discussion useful. Parts of it are summarized below. First, by using secondary analysis, full use can be made of these existing data that were very expensive (in terms of money and researchers' and subjects' time) to collect. Some large-scale data sets can be useful for addressing macrolevel hypotheses that would be prohibitively expensive to address at multiple sites. Follow-ups can be done of subjects in what were originally conceived as cross-sectional studies, instead of doing time-consuming longitudinal research from the beginning. Existing data sets can be used to replicate and extend prior findings. Replication, a basic tenet of science and a particularly important one in a field with social policy implications, is rare, so existing data sets should add considerable value to the field of family research. Similarly, exploratory hypotheses, difficult to test when they depend on the execution of a major undertaking, can be tested on an existing data set and be used in guiding future research design.

Next, secondary analysis can be very useful in mapping social change by comparing findings from similar or identical studies conducted at various points in history. For example, Johnson and Booth (1990) studied the relation between marital quality, mental health, and economic distress in a group of Nebraska farmers during a period of farm hardship in the late 1970s and early 1980s. They compared their findings with those reported in another secondary analysis of a similar topic: Liker and Elder's (1983) study of marital relations and economic hardship during the Great Depression. Generally, similar relationships were found, although some of Liker and Elder's specific findings were not replicated in the Johnson and Booth study. Methodological differences cannot be separated from cohort differences in these two studies, underscoring the value of secondary analyses that involve identical methods at different points in history.

Finally, Colby notes that, as a companion to collecting data concerning new theories, it is often useful to reanalyze existing data using these new theories. For example, researchers interested in examining the relevance for females of theories now seen as "male-centered" could both collect new data based on new formulations of the problem and reanalyze older data using coding schemes from the new theory. In this way, differences found between the newer and older studies can be interpreted as being due to theoretical versus cohort differences.

PROBLEMS WITH SECONDARY ANALYSIS

Of course, there are also potential problems inherent in this practice of reanalyzing existing data. The overarching problem is that the data may imperfectly fit the needs of the secondary analyst. Specifically, the theory or model that drove the original research will have influenced every level of the original data collection (e.g., how the sample was drawn, what was asked, how it was asked, how the responses were coded). Even the meaning of a particular question may change over time. Consider an imaginary data set from a study of day-care versus home-reared infants' attachment to mothers that was collected in the 1970s. It would have been quite appropriate and theoretically consistent for researchers interested in this topic to interview mothers about their babies' attachment to them and to film the reactions of the infants when their mothers left the room. At first glance, the data might seem ripe for reanalysis by researchers in the 1990s interested in the reciprocity of infant and maternal attachment (that is, the mutual attachment of infant to mother and mother to infant). But there are many pitfalls here. First, children in day care in the 1990s and in the 1970s probably had mothers with different demographic profiles, so conclusions about current mother-infant pairs might be suspect. Second, because of the prevalent theories about attachment at the time, the 1970s interviews would probably have focused on the baby's behavior and/or apparent emotions around attachment issues to the exclusion of questions about mothers' behavior and emotions, so that it is possible that half of the current model cannot be addressed. Third, some of the questions asked might have a different meaning in 1990 than in the 1970s (e.g., "How does your baby react when you leave him?" might have a different meaning to women whose husbands are equal sharers in child-rearing and/or to women who have left their children in the care of others often, so, again, conclusions about current cohorts would be risky). And, finally, the 1970s films would probably have focused only on the mother-infant pair (as opposed to including fathers, as current models of family process might recommend), and mostly on the infant at that (and the researchers might even have instructed all mothers to behave in some constant way), instead of focusing in addition on mothers' behavior during the interaction. Even if there had been one or two questions related to mothers' perceptions, or a few moments of observation of the mothers on the films, the input about the mother would probably be thin (therefore conclusions about the relative impact on the dyadic relationship of the mother and infant might be misleading).

Several other problems with secondary analysis may exist as well. First, the psychometric properties of archival data may not be known. In some cases, excellent psychometric manuals accompany archival data, or the primary and secondary analysts can confer on these matters, but the reliability and validity of the scores must be addressed anew. Similarly, sometimes the archival data include the final coding scores of interview or observational data. The secondary analyst who just wants to use these scores at least needs to know how the coding was done so she/he can make sense of the results, and this coding information may not be fully available. Secondary analysts who want to compare these coding scores with scores from other studies using the same coding system must have access to raw data from all studies and make sure that the current coders are reliable with the original coding.

Another problem is that the available data may be aggregated in ways that interfere with a reliable and valid test of a hypothesis about the functioning of individuals or families. The secondary analyst must be particularly alert to the dangers of making cross-level inferences. For example, if a data set provides mean scores on such variables as education, unemployment, child-rearing values, and reported cases of family violence by school district, then the researcher is not automatically justified in drawing inferences about the relationships between these variables at the level of individuals or families. That is to say, with school district being the unit of analysis, one might find a positive association between education and preference for democratic child-rearing styles. One would not, however, be correct to assume that within a particular district, the higher the education of the parents, the stronger the preference for democratic practices. Although such a positive relation might exist across the full range of scores from the various school districts, within any one district, where the range might be quite small, the relation could be zero or even negative (see Pedhazur, 1982, for a discussion of this issue of cross-level inference).

Thus there are challenges that may arise with secondary analysis, many of which are problems that can be fixed while the others may be tolerable as long as they are recognized. See Box 5.1 for an example of problems that arose in some investigators' secondary analysis of their own data. In short, a very clear understanding of the sample characteristics, data collection procedures, coding methods, and data analysis decisions is critical before embarking on any secondary analysis.

FAMILY AND SOCIAL ARCHIVES AND DOCUMENTS

What about the "data" that families and societies keep about and for themselves? Family archives (e.g., family photo albums, home movies, or letters, in which family members portray themselves, not for a researcher, but for their own purposes) and social archives (child-rearing advice books, magazine articles, and textbooks, in which current social values are revealed) may more realistically tell us about family issues than data collected in a research study. The use of unobtrusive measures like these has not been common in family research, but could be quite fruitful (see Webb et al., 1966).

Blinn (1988), for example, coded sets of 100 family photographs from a sample of families. She compared her coding of the photos (along dimensions of cohesiveness, expressiveness, conflict, independence, achievement, intellectual/cultural, activity/recreational, moral/religious, outdoor/nature, and time/history) with raters' and family members' ratings on these same dimensions and with family members' scores on the Family Environment Scale. The photo coding was correlated with family self-ratings, particularly those of the wives.

BOX 5.1
Using Previously Collected Data to Ask New Questions

Using interviews with mothers and children collected during a study of parental divorce, Copeland, Stewart, and Healy (1989) were able to address questions about the "parentification" of children in the study. Parentification is a term coined by family therapists to refer to the process of having children in a family take on adult- or "parent"-like roles. Children who worry about whether there's enough money to pay the bills, or who are responsible for waking their mothers up in the morning, for example, are said to be parentified, and may be at some risk for developing some kinds of problems.

The divorce study was designed using traditional developmental and personality theories and methods, so trying to score a family-systems construct like parentification raised a number of issues common to many secondary analyses:

1. *The interview questions available for recoding were not exactly the ones that we would have asked had we been primarily interested in parentification while designing the study.* Because the questions driving the original study had to do with individual outcome and overall adjustment at the time of parental separation, the interview questions centered on issues of daily life, history of marriage and separation, and feelings about the separation. While the answers to these questions provided a rich source of information about family life in which issues of parentification often arose, were we to design a study specifically on this issue we would have asked specifically about parentification.

2. *We did not have full reports about all family members from all family members, as would have been preferred in a study of family process.* Mothers and one child, age 6 to 12, were the focus of the study, although interviews were also held with the other children and, when possible, fathers. Complete information about adjustment and divorce reaction was available only on the one randomly chosen "target" child, and, even in families with parentification issues, that target child may or may not have been the parentified one in the family. Thus in some analyses, we restricted our focus to those measures available for all children; in others, we used just those target children who were parentified and in so doing had a smaller sample of parentified children than was probably truly represented in the whole study.

3. *The study design restricted the generalizability of the results.* All the families in the study were undergoing parental separation, so we were only able to learn about parentification in separating families. In fact, this was, in itself, a very relevant consideration because family process during major transformations is quite important to understand. However, in a study designed specifically to understand this family dynamic, we might have included a nonseparating group.

Family photos will also be the main data source in a study of the lives of Mississippi blacks, conducted by the Center for the Study of Southern Culture at the University of Mississippi and the Duke University Center for Documentary Studies (*Chronicle of Higher Education*, February 21, 1990). The goal will be to provide an insider's account of black familes in Mississippi as a balance to the predominance of outsiders' accounts that focus on politics and struggles.

Important information about the early mother-infant interactions of autistic children has been obtained by studying home movies of families in which the infant, nondiagnosed at the time of the movie, was later diagnosed as psychotic or autistic. Thus the films allowed a prospective-like study of severe disturbance. Massie (1978, 1980) was able to describe the constitutional qualities of young infants, their neuromuscular pathology, initial signs of pathology, and maternal-infant interaction in 10 infants who were diagnosed as psychotic or autistic several years after the films were taken. Disturbances in both mothers' behavior (e.g., avoidance of eye contact, brusqueness, insensitivity) and infants' behavior (e.g., less-than-normal activity, delays in motor development, disinterest in objects and people) were found.

Wrightsman (1981) describes the potential benefits of analyzing personal documents (such as diaries, letters, autobiographies, and memoirs) to study adult personality development. He reviews several studies of personal documents, including several that concern family-related issues like separation anxiety (Sears, 1979) and the mother-son relationship (Allport, 1965). Stewart, Franz, and Layton (1988) studied the individual life of Vera Brittain, a British feminist and pacifist who was a young adult at the time of World War I. Using Erikson's theory of personality development, they coded expressions of preoccupation with aspects of identity, intimacy, and generativity found in her diaries, letters, and autobiography, all personal documents produced for purposes other than research.

At a sociocultural level of analysis of the family, Bryant and Coleman (1988) reviewed 25 marriage and family textbooks, published between 1980 and 1987, for content about black familes. In order to locate material on black familes, they looked in tables of contents and indexes for key words (e.g., blacks, Afro-Americans, Negroes, minorities, interracial marriage). On the basis of the number of pages devoted to black families, they categorized texts in terms of the predominant perspective toward black families: 9 were coded as deviance oriented (in which black families were discussed only under topics implying dysfunction, such as welfare or divorce) and 13 as culturally equivalent (in which black families were discussed under categories not implying dysfunction, and differences between black and white families were attributed to causes other than race). Three were coded as mixed. None considered the black family within the context of its own history and sociopolitical milieu (the cultural variant perspective).

STRENGTHS AND LIMITATIONS OF STUDYING FAMILY AND SOCIAL DOCUMENTS

The obvious strength of this approach to the study of families is that the researcher is allowed a glimpse at family life that has been otherwise kept out of the domain of science. The portrayal of the families, unimpeded by demand characteristics (i.e., the families are trying to please the researcher or to respond in the way they think is expected of them), can be very exciting. And, as in the case of the home movies of the autistic/psychotic children, family documents can allow a type of prospective research design.

There are also certain problems with using family and social documents, however. First, the validity of the information about the family needs serious attention but may be difficult to assess. Does the information gleaned really mean what the researcher thinks it means? Is it a full description of the family on that dimension? For example, the Blinn (1988) paper cited earlier reported low agreement between the photograph coding and the family's report on a widely used self-report family measure, but would we necessarily expect that the two approaches would yield similar descriptions of the families? And one could question how accurately textbook and magazine writers reflect real, broad social values about families.

Second, sampling issues, a concern for all researchers, may be particularly germane here. Webb et al. (1966) mention "selective deposit" and "selective survival" issues. Are families that produce ("deposit") family archive material different from those who do not do so? Are families that keep material around over the years different from those who throw it away ("survival")? Further, what are the characteristics of families that have over 100 family photographs on hand? Are they particularly self-conscious? Particularly attractive? Particularly family oriented? What about those who have and use a video or movie camera? Are they particularly rich? Unusually theatrical or self-confident? And those who write a lot of letters to each other—are they particularly verbal and fluent? Shy? Too poor to afford telephone calls? And why are they apart from those to whom they are writing? Obviously, there are good answers to many of these questions within the particular domains of some research topics, but they are questions that should be raised in doing this kind of research.

EXERCISE

1. Explore Webb's et al. (1966) notion of the running record by trying to make a list of *all* institutions, agencies, or businesses that have some record on you, going back to the time you were born. For example, include schools, doctors and hospitals, credit agencies, and political organizations. Which of these might lend themselves to interesting family-research questions, if proper informed consent for access could be obtained?

RECOMMENDED READING

Colby, A. (1982). The use of secondary analysis in the study of women and social change. *Journal of Social Issues, 38*(1), 119-123.
Stewart, D. W. (1984). *Secondary research: Information sources and methods.* Beverly Hills, CA: Sage.
Webb, E. J., Campbell, D. T., Schwartz, R. D., & Sechrest, L. (1966). *Nonreactive research in the social sciences.* Boston: Houghton Mifflin.
Wrightsman, L. S. (1981). Personal documents as data in conceptualizing adult personality development. *Personality and Social Psychology Bulletin, 7*(3), 367-385.

6

Quantitative Data Analysis

Once the data have been collected and coded, whether in the form of questionnaires, survey results, or coded observations, some degree of quantification usually is done in order for data analysis to proceed (however, refer to the section on qualitative analysis in Chapter 2 for a different approach). To some extent, the techniques of data reduction and analysis used in family research studies are the same as, or at least based on, those used in traditional psychological research. A number of issues arise that make traditional data analysis approaches less useful, however, when one tries to describe whole groups, to combine several people's scores into one family measure, or to capture sequences of observed interactions between family members. In this chapter, the special problems faced by family researchers in their attempts to interpret the collected data are described.

THE NONINDEPENDENCE ISSUE

In traditional psychological research, data are collected for individual subjects of various types who are then compared with each other. Most statistical methods were developed to handle data (questionnaire responses, test scores, behavioral codes) from single individuals who are completely independent from the other individuals in the study. And most tests of significance presume that the subjects involved in a study have been randomly sampled from the population of interest. Obviously, this assumption is violated when members of the same family are involved, and this causes a number of problems. For one clear example of how this violation can be problematic, consider a study of the effects of fathers' child-rearing strategies on children's achievement orientation. We might ask whether fathers who are very strict about school and discipline have children who get higher grades and are more driven to succeed than more laid-back fathers. It would pose special statistical issues to include two children from each family because the children in each family share the same father. In effect, each father's child-rearing strategy would get "counted" twice, even though he was only one father.

If one father happened to be extreme in some child-rearing behavior and his two children happened to be extreme (either very high or very low) in achievement orientation, the results might unfairly suggest that that particular parental behavior was more important than it really was. Thus it has traditionally been a statistical requirement that subjects in a study be completely independent of each other. A traditional solution to this problem would be to select randomly one child from each study family and to study the behavior of each father and target child, ignoring the other children.

In family research, of course, the requirement of statistical independence, by definition, is often not met and the traditional solutions are unsatisfactory. Many questions of concern to family researchers dictate the collection of data from or about more than one person per family; for example, how and why siblings are different from each other, how spouses' attitudes or behaviors compare, or how parents versus children perceive the importance of particular family traits. Some researchers have suggested that if one can assume, either on empirical or theoretical grounds, that family factor variance (i.e., variance in scores attributable to respondents being in the same family) is very low, no special provision has to be made in the statistical comparison of family members' scores (Schumm, Barnes, Bollman, Jurich, & Milliken, 1984). More generally, most researchers assume that family factor variance may always be present, and try to take account of it statistically. Where the goal is to compare two or more people within a family, there are statistics designed for correlated samples, usually modifications of statistics for independent groups, designed to handle nonindependent data:

(1) *Nonindependent* t *test.* Suppose you were interested in whether mothers and fathers had different patterns of attachment to their last-born children. (For example, in the family of David and Nancy, discussed in Chapter 1, one might have asked this question, given the current closeness of David and Natalie, and the distance of Nancy from both.) You could collect some measure of attachment from each parent. But since the parents would each be rating their relationship to the same child (who has a given set of temperament, physical, and behavioral traits that might influence attachment), you would not want to consider your sample as being simply a group of unrelated men and women. Instead of a simple *t* test, then, a better choice might be a variation of it, a *t* test for nonindependent groups, in which the dependent variable was a pair of scores, one from each parent in a given family. White et al. (1986) used this statistic in their study of their intimacy maturity

to demonstrate that husbands and wives did not differ significantly from each other in intimacy and marital adjustment scores.

(2) *Repeated measures analysis of variance.* Similarly, suppose you had more than two levels of a particular factor (e.g., if you were interested in comparing the reactions of mothers, fathers, and adolescents to some family trauma like a house fire). Rather than using a simple one-way analysis of variance (ANOVA), a better choice would be to account for the probable family factor variance (the mothers, fathers, and adolescents in a family shared an experience that is likely to be different in both subtle and explicit ways from the experience of other families undergoing a house fire) and use a repeated measures ANOVA. Here, the dependent variable would be the mother's, father's, and adolescent's fire reaction. This method also allows the inclusion of several factors. For example, you also might want to include a between-groups factor like "availability of family support following trauma" to the above analyses. Then your questions could be as follows:

(a) Do mothers, fathers, and children differ in their reactions to traumatic fires? (main effect for Family Member, a repeated measures factor)
(b) Does having family support nearby alleviate the stress of the trauma? (main effect for Family Support, not a repeated measures factor since whole families either had or did not have support)
(c) Does having family support nearby affect mothers, fathers, and adolescents differentially? (interaction of factors)

(3) *Multiple regression.* In a multiple regression analysis, family members' individual scores on some variable are entered into an equation to try to predict some criterion score. For example, are the job satisfaction ratings of mothers and fathers related to their child's school performance? Or, in the study involving David and Nancy, one might ask whether mothers' and/or fathers' early memories of their own childhood families predict the current level of family cohesion. Using multiple regression, one could learn whether mothers' or fathers' job satisfaction/early memory scores were more consistently related to child or family outcome, and, if so, whether the other spouse's ratings contributed additional important information. This procedure is useful except when scores of family members are highly correlated with each other.

THE LEVEL OF
VARIABLE FORMATION ISSUE

In other cases, the concern is not so much to compare people within a family as to capture some sense of the family as a whole, or to quantify into a single variable the data from several family members so that families can be compared with each other. (This issue is the same if one is interested in subsystems rather than whole families.) For example, "What is the relationship between parental alcoholism and the family's level of functioning in the community?" "What happens to an immigrating family's sense of cohesion as it encounters a new culture?" or "What is the effect of being in an earthquake on a family's sense of control and safety?" Here, families, not individuals, form the unit of analysis. That is to say, each family, not each person, should have a score—a score of the family's level of functioning, the family's level of cohesion, or the family's sense of control and safety. The problem is in coming up with a score that accurately describes the whole family when the actual data have been collected from each family member individually, or, to use the term introduced in Chapter 2, to form the variables at a family level. What if people within a single family differ on the construct of interest—maybe one person reports feeling quite safe and another quite unsafe. What if people within a family disagree on how they view things—maybe one person in a family thinks the father has a drinking problem and another person does not.

Of course, there are some important questions of concern to family researchers in which one individual's score may be adequate, even thorough. These may include studies relying on self-report or individual behavior scores (e.g., "What is the course of women's marital satisfaction following the birth of a first child?"), or on individuals' reports about other family members (e.g., "Are young adults' descriptions of their relationships with their parents related to their descriptions of their relationships with their own children?"). In other cases, the data as originally collected may already refer to the group as a whole (e.g., "Is the speed with which a family solves a laboratory problem related in a meaningful way to their perceptions of control?"). For example, Bennett, Wolin, Reiss, and Teitelbaum (1987) interviewed couples together in a study of family history and alcoholism. The researchers gave scores to the couples as a whole, not to each member of a couple, so that there was no collapsing of data to be done—each score already "belonged" only to the couple. In these cases, one could comfortably dismiss the unit of analysis issue.

The first question a researcher should ask, then, is whether trying to derive a whole-family score from data from individual members is necessary and makes sense. Perhaps it is not warranted by the research question, or perhaps it would involve collapsing of the data across family members, with the danger that doing so will mask important information. Perhaps it would be better to choose one person randomly and focus on her or him. While this is certainly a possibility, some family researchers often try to accommodate, indeed capture, the complexity inherent in intrafamily disagreement. For example, one might argue that in studying the parental alcoholism/family mental health question, one would most sensibly just randomly pick one child per alcoholic family and study his or her mental health. If just one child per family were included, the data would satisfy the independence criterion for most statistical analyses, and some important questions about alcoholism could be addressed. Indeed, the great bulk of psychological research has taken this defensible position. But would it not also be important to know if all the children in a family usually responded similarly to each other? Or whether there tended to be a wide range of reaction, some children having few problems, others showing a lot of negative response? These are not better questions, simply different questions than have typically been asked before.

There are a number of questions to consider when deciding how to derive a family score from individually collected data. The answers to these questions will influence the choice of method of score development.

1. Is the (inevitable) disagreement among family members considered simply measurement error, or is it interesting information in itself? That is to say, there are some topics where one could assume there is some more or less "true" answer, though family members may differ as to how accurately they report it (for example, "How long has your father been unemployed?" or "How long has the marital conflict been going on?"). Even here, in some cases individual members' deviation from the "accurate" answer might be seen as valuable information. In others, there is no assumption that one person's view is more accurate than another's ("How happy is your marriage?").

2. Are there some members of the family who are likely to have more accurate perceptions than other members, and whose reports, therefore, should be given more weight, or is everyone's report equally germane? In asking about the history of marital conflict, for example, each spouse's report

might be seen as more valid than that of any of the children. But in asking about reactions to trauma, each person's self-report might be considered equally relevant.

3. Who is considered the best source of information about the family? In the case where the focus is on one individual's outcome, for example, is that individual's phenomenological self-report of the outcome variable the most, or indeed the only, valid indicator of outcome, or are the views of the other family members also relevant? If one is examining the role of some family variable in affecting that individual's outcome, should the rating of the family variable be done simply by that individual, or is the collective sense of the family more valid? Even if the family combined score is considered more "real," is that score truly more important to the outcome than the individual's perception of the family?

4. Are there equivalent data from each member, or is one person's contribution to an aggregated score likely to have disproportionate weight? For example, if each member of a divorcing family is asked to review the history of the family and marriage, the parents probably would give much longer and more detailed answers than would the children. If these answers were then coded for number of indications of anger, the parents might have higher scores simply because they talked longer. Obviously, one would not want to conclude from this method that the parents were more angry than the children. Just how differential weighting is done is quite a complicated matter, however. There are a number of options, each with substantially different conceptual outcomes. Say the number of children in the families in a given study was different, for example. One could give every child in a family a certain weight, letting each child carry an equivalent input, but making the input of "the children" larger in bigger families. Or one could establish a "children's contribution," some summary of all the children's input combined, and use that score instead.

There is no "right" way to answer these questions. Rather, the decisions about how to interpret input from different family members must be consistent with the theory driving the research and used in defining the constructs. The researcher needs to consider the conceptual effect a particular decision will have on the meaning of the data analyses.

For example, a number of solutions to the problem of deriving family scores based on individual data have been developed by family researchers. The best solution depends on the answers to the questions listed above, and the researcher's weighing of the advantages and disadvantages of the statistical properties of each solution. Fisher et al. (1985) provide a useful review of many options, along with a discussion of the limitations of each (the interested reader is urged to read their article carefully. The options noted by these authors are summarized as follows:

(1) *Using the family mean.* When several individuals in a family are asked to rate a particular construct, one option is to find the arithmetic mean of the individuals' scores as a way to describe the family's score on that construct. For example, Sigafoos et al. (1985) asked each family member to complete the FACES measure of cohesion and adaptability. One of the measures the authors used in their analyses was the mean across all members on this scale. While this is clearly a convenient and conceptually simple measure, it is not always the measure of choice. A mean score hides the level of intrafamilial disagreement (e.g., a mean score of 50 could be obtained by a family with scores of 49, 50, and 51, or by a family with scores of 10, 50, and 90). If deviance in scores within a family is of conceptual interest to the researcher, it would be a mistake to use a family mean of individual scores; the deviant scores would become camouflaged by the mean. And it is important to note that in a mean score, each family member contributes equally to the score; sometimes this is desirable, but sometimes it is not. Research on marital satisfaction, for example, might include higher, even if not exclusive, weighting of the parents' ratings relative to the children's. Finally, it is important to recognize that in using a family mean, you are saying that that mean score is an adequate substitute for each individual score. Thus it should be established that the various individuals' scores are positively correlated with each other, preferably highly, whenever a mean score is used.

(2) *Using a "nonredundant sum" across family members.* If every family in a sample has the same number of participating members, using a simple sum of scores across members is equivalent to using a mean. Comments about the limitations of mean scores would apply here as well. A variation of this, however, includes using a "nonredundant sum" (Fisher et al., 1985), a score particularly useful for recording the occurrence of discrete events. All family members might be asked to rate whether a list of events (such as life events, school visits, or marital disputes) happened. Then the researcher would count in the family score any event that any family member rated as having occurred, disregarding family disagreement.

(3) *Using extreme scores only.* Some investigators argue that one person in a family holding an extreme view in fact always influences the family as a whole, even if the other members report more moderate views. For example, Klein and Hill (1979) asked family members to rate their satisfaction with their family's solution in a problem-solving

task. The data point used in the analysis, rather than the sum or mean of the satisfaction ratings, was the rating of the least satisfied member. Obviously, this method carries with it some important theoretical assumptions about how families work, assumptions that would have to be met any time the method was used.

(4) *Using difference scores.* Often, family researchers are interested in how much family members agree with each other about a particular topic. Disagreement itself (almost regardless of the topic) has been thought to be indicative of certain types of family stress. (Consider the old marital complaint, "If I say it's white, he says it's black.") Thus one quantitative indicator of family discord is sometimes taken to be the difference between members' ratings. For example, parents might be asked to rate their child on dimensions of cooperativeness, flexibility, and responsiveness; highly discrepant scores between parents rating the same child would certainly seem to be a meaningful piece of data about the child's role in that family. One problem with this method, though, is that a difference score (e.g., husband's score minus the wife's score) loses all information about the relative level of their ratings. The difference between 90 and 100 is the same as the difference between 1 and 11; are couples with these pairs of scores truly comparable? It may be that the answer to this question is "yes," depending on the construct being measured and the theory that drives the study, but this has to be clear from the beginning. In addition, in the case where the two scores in question are positively correlated (the probable case in such family research) difference scores tend to be less reliable than the individual scores involved (i.e., the percent of error variance is increased). It is harder to reach statistical significance with unreliable scores due to this loss in power. Thus before using a difference score, you would want to establish that the individual scores involved in the subtraction are, themselves, quite reliable.

Taking a slightly different approach to the question of disagreement scores, Szinovacz (1983) administered the Straus (1979) Conflict Tactics Scale (to measure marital violence) to husbands and wives and computed two *agreement* scores: the total agreement ratio (whether couples agreed either that violence did occur between them *or* that violence did not occur) and the violence agreement ratio (of those couples in which at least one spouse reported violence, the proportion of those in which both spouses reported it). While this approach avoided some of the problems of difference scores, it collapsed the data across "type of violence" and amount of violence reported, and thus is quite a rough estimate of violence in the family.

(5) *Combining level and discrepancy information statistically.* Obviously, there are attractive features in each of the above methods of making a family-level score from individuals' data, and it sometimes seems a shame to have to choose one to the exclusion of another. One option is to control statistically for one score while focusing primarily on another, (e.g., one could use a difference score in an analysis, with a couple mean score as a covariate.) Multiple regression analysis could also be used, entering a couple mean level score and the spouse discrepancy score into the equation to try to predict some criterion score. An empirical, though atheoretical, answer to the question of the primacy of importance of these scores would thus be obtained. Indeed, whether a particular family outcome is best predicted by a summary versus a discrepancy score can be quite a provocative and theoretically interesting question. Finally, one could sacrifice some of the information available in each family member's continuous score and make a sort of typology. For example, families could be divided along two dimensions: high, medium, or low husband's score; and high, medium, or low wife's score. Each family, then, would be roughly classified according to both level and spousal agreement. As before, the choice among these methods depends on your assessment of the ways in which statistical and theoretical assumptions are being met in your study.

(6) *Using cluster analysis.* Another approach to understanding how families compare with each other is to use the multivariate approach of cluster analysis (Filsinger, 1990). Here, individual family members' scores on a given variable are entered into an analysis, and clusters, or groupings, of families, based on intrafamily similarity, are produced. This approach has been especially useful at the theory-building or hypothesis-forming stage since, in fact, the clusters that are formed are made purely empirically, not on the basis of a hypothesis.

The meaning and relationship among some of these types of scores are discussed, using data from a family research study, by Larsen and Olson (1990). Of course, this is not a complete list of all the options available to family researchers for forming family-level scores from individual data. One can creatively combine one's knowledge of the theory or assumptions driving the research with one's understanding of the properties of various statistics to form the best, possibly new, solution. For example, Walters, Pittman, and Norrel (1984) used a technique called communality analysis. Here, the unique variance accounted for by each family member in predicting the total family sum on each item of a questionnaire was used to weight the absolute level of each individual's questionnaire total score. It would, of course, be possible, using this approach, also to include the variance accounted for by a particular dyad in the family as a weight. Again, one simply has to recognize the conceptual assumptions being made when using a particular method of combining or weighting individual scores. As Walters and colleagues (1984) noted, "Initially the statistical treatment appears complex, but once it is grasped, it is apparent that the more complex issue is in the conceptualization of families."

THE MOVING PICTURE ISSUE

Family researchers who use observational methods often face another problem if they are interested in capturing something about the *sequence* of interactions that occur. Many traditional observational coding systems involve a simple count or sum of ratings of a number of behaviors that occur during an observation; for example, the number of times a husband criticizes his wife, or the number of maternal commands a child obeys. These counts are certainly useful and important, but they tell little about "what happened, and then what happened next." Does the child tend to disobey the mother following paternal criticism of the mother? Or does the father tend to criticize the mother after the child disobeys? Or does the father's criticism of the mother function to increase the number of commands the mother gives to the child, increasing the probability that the child will disobey some of them? Simple counts of criticisms, commands, and failures to obey cannot answer these questions. As Hinde (1979) notes, whether a couple usually kisses after they quarrel or usually quarrels after they kiss is quite an important distinction, although the overall rates of kissing and quarreling may be the same!

One method of analyzing some types of observational data—*sequential analysis*—allows these "what-happens-next" questions to be addressed. While certainly not used exclusively by family researchers, sequential analysis has become an important tool for understanding family process. (See Bakeman & Gottman, 1986, for an introduction to and step-by-step description of sequential analysis, and Cousins & Power, 1986, for a discussion of some of the issues that have arisen in the use of this technique in family research.)

As a brief example of sequential analysis, assume there are four verbal categories in a given simple code system (A = Mother asks question, B = Child asks question, C = Mother responds, and D = Child responds). A conversation might go like this: ADADADBCBDBCAD (Mother Asks Question-Child Responds-Mother Asks Question, and so forth). Sequential analysis allows one to ask, "How often does a child's question get answered by the mother (how often does the B-C sequence occur), and is this higher than one would expect by chance?"

Sequential analysis, then, is a method of capturing real sequences of behavior, rather than static counts or numbers. It also is useful in uncovering less obvious sequences, such as those separated by time or intervening behavior. For example, take the case in which the father's criticism of the mother functions to increase the number of commands the mother gives to the child. Maybe this does in fact happen, but not immediately. Perhaps the increase in commands reliably comes within a few minutes, but is not necessarily the very next thing the mother says following receiving a criticism. This is, in fact, likely, since people are not automatons, but rather take time to process their feelings, or take the eggs off the stove(!) before they respond. Thus a method is needed that will record reliable sequences that are not necessarily adjacent in time. A special kind of sequential analysis—lag sequential analysis—can do that.

Lag sequential analysis offers another benefit to observational researchers. It can reveal the likelihood of two 2-event sequences occurring together. Continuing the example above, perhaps the father's criticism of the mother is usually prompted by the child's disobeying. Then, in fact, what really seems to happen in this family is that, for some reason or another, Child Disobeys-Father Criticizes Mother, then (perhaps immediately, perhaps after some time) Mother Commands-Child Disobeys. The probability of these two 2-event sequences co-occurring can be calculated using lag sequential analysis procedures. The possibilities for starting to capture some of the circularity and complexity of the family process become clear.

Of course, trying to code every act in a long observation can be extremely time consuming. Perhaps it is only the behavior that surrounds a particular type of incident that is of interest. For example, Vuchinich, Emery, and Cassidy (1988) were interested in the role that third parties played in dyadic family conflict—do other family members intervene to mediate, distract, or prolong a conflict that started between two people? These researchers recorded 52 families at dinnertime; the tapes were reviewed by coders for instances of verbal conflict. Analysis of various types of sequences was then conducted on these conflict instances only.

While a thorough description of sequential analysis is beyond the scope of this book, the basic steps can be described in order to relay a sense of the procedure.

- First, one puts the data into event or time series form. To continue the four-code example of mothers' and children's questions and responses used earlier, one might have a sequence of simple behaviors like this: ADADADBCBDBCAD
- Then, one computes the simple and transitional probabilities of the behaviors of interest. The simple probability of Mother Responds (code C in this example) refers to the proportion of total events that were coded as Mother Responds (i.e., total number of Cs [2] divided by the total number of events in the sequence [14], or .143). A transitional probability is slightly more complex and more informative. It refers to the probability of one event occurring, given the occurrence of another event—for example, of Mother Responds occurring, given the number of times Child Asks Question. Here, the behavior, Child Asks Questions (code B) occurred three times and the sequence Child Asks Question-Mother Responds (codes B-C) twice. The transitional probability, then, is 2 (number of B-C sequences) divided by 3 (total number of code Bs), or .666.
- Finally, one is interested in whether the level of these probability scores is higher than what would be expected by chance. One can determine the statistical significance by the use of the z score, or the chi-square goodness of fit test, both of which address the question, "Is what was observed significantly different from what was expected by chance?"

Note that sequential analysis is not a method of coding observations, but rather of analyzing already-coded observational data. Some types of observational code procedures allow the use of this procedure, and some do not. The following conditions must be met before this is an appropriate technique:

First, it is important that every bit of behavior in a given interaction series has been coded in the order it occurred, as is true in an event-sampling procedure. This is so because one wants to assess "what-follows-what." In simple tally or timing methods, one has lost all information about the order in which various behaviors happened. In time-sampling methods, one might not have coded this entire sequence.

In addition to being exhaustive, the coding categories must be mutually exclusive; a given act cannot be coded into two categories. For example, if a person smiled while asking a question, and both the smile and the question were deemed important by the researcher, there would have to be a separate code, "Asks question while smiling."

Third, there must be enough data points (events in the sequence) to allow for testing of significance. Obviously, if you just watched a dyad or family for 30 seconds and got 7 coded behaviors, it would be impossible to infer anything about the real probability of a particular sequence! But how long is long enough? Siegel (1956) suggests a criterion of:

$$NP(1 - P) \geq 9$$

where P = expected probability of a particular sequence and N = total number of sequences categorized.

Sequential analysis holds much promise for coders of observations of families because of its utility in capturing the "action" of family relationships. The interested reader is strongly urged to read further about this approach, starting with the introductory book by Bakeman and Gottman (1986).

USING STATISTICS TO CAPTURE THE COMPLEXITY AND DYNAMISM OF THE FAMILY

Many—perhaps most—statistical procedures used by family researchers are largely grounded in individual psychology and will not get a detailed representation here. Solving the unit of analysis problem and nonindependence issues discussed earlier in this chapter paves the way for family researchers to use more generic statistical procedures. Because of the predicted complexity of family relationships in many of the theories, though, family researchers tend to use statistical approaches that can handle multiple variables and discern complex interactions. The reader should consult any basic social science statistics book for a description of each test. Basically, family researchers often

- want to describe the frequency of some phenomenon, and use descriptive statistics to do so;
- have simple or linear hypotheses involving two variables at a time, and use correlation, t tests, or analysis of variance to test them;
- have nonlinear hypotheses and use polynomial regression to test them;
- have hypotheses involving more than two variables at a time and use multivariate statistics, like multiple regression, multivariate analysis of variance, logistic regression, factor analysis, cluster analysis, or discriminant analysis, to test them; or

- want to examine indirect effects or moderator variables, each with a single indicator, where all effects are hypothesized to be unidirectional, and use path analysis to do so.

Although most quantitative family researchers to date have successfully relied on these kinds of basic statistics, there is a growing reluctance among many family researchers to continue using models of family process that are simple, linear, and formulated on the basis of available techniques of analysis. Certainly, the foundation for all family research lies in research that has investigated the broad strokes, main effects, and simple interactions, and certainly more of this research needs to be done. But we now know enough about a multitude of factors that influence family interaction that we could start to put many of these into single models.

Such models would include several, even many, constructs simultaneously. Perhaps each construct would best be measured by a number of variables, and perhaps these variables would have different types of relationships to each other (e.g., some linear, some nonlinear). Further, some variables in the model might be related to each other in a unidirectional causal way, with others related in a reciprocal fashion.

Rather than look at some simple direct relationship between two factors, we are interested in trying to incorporate more and more influences into a given model. For example, rather than a simple focus on the effect of parental discipline strategies on adolescents' delinquency, we might want to include such factors as the effect of the adolescents' misbehavior on parental discipline strategies; the role of sibling behavior on both the target adolescent and the parents; the parents' own experience with and expectations about parental discipline; and the influence of marital friction on the family (i.e., on the adolescent, on the parents themselves, on siblings, or on other people who in turn might affect the discipline-delinquency relationship). Several points are important here. One is that the complexity of all these relationships is difficult to capture. The other is that some of the influences that we suspect are critical and in fact precede (in some cases by moments, in other cases by many years) any observed causal relationship between parental discipline and adolescent delinquency. Also of importance, we know that adolescent misbehavior itself is sure to influence the next parental discipline encounter.

Even though statistical tests for this kind of model are beginning to be available, they often involve assumptions and requirements that are still very difficult for family researchers to meet (see Godwin, 1988, for a discussion of the use of structural equation modeling in family research). For example, to use structural equation modeling (an approach to testing a model with many predictors, each of which may have been measured by several methods, and which may include reciprocal and/or nonlinear relationships with the outcome variable), the researcher must be sure that *all* relevant variables in the prediction of an outcome have been included and measured. But how often are we sure we have not missed an important influence? And if we are pretty sure, don't we often end up with a very large number of influences? Second, a researcher using structural equation modeling must be sure to have specified in advance, on theoretical grounds, the nature (e.g., direction, shape, size) of the expected relationships between variables in the model. Family theory and empirical literature may not be able to support such precise predictions.

There are also stringent assumptions regarding sample size, design, and data distribution that must be met before structural equation modeling is an appropriate choice. Family researchers are likely to be including many parameters (especially given the requirement that the model be theoretically complete), and at least some of the constructs are likely to have been measured in time- and money-intensive ways, putting the brakes on how many subjects can be easily obtained. Even when all these difficult conditions have been met, assumptions of causality must be made very cautiously (Biddle & Marlin, 1987; Godwin, 1988; J. A. Martin, 1987). These limitations are certainly not a fault of the statistical approach, but rather pose a promising challenge to family researchers that if they can develop and collect the right kind of data, statisticians can test their models very well.

To reiterate, then, the foundation for statistical solutions for these problems is established, with the development of multivariate statistics, and various modeling techniques, though these techniques often require statistical and theoretical assumptions that family researchers cannot make. Further, many of these techniques are not yet readily accessible to most family researchers. The November 1988 issue of *Journal of Marriage and the Family,* the February 1987 issue of *Child Development,* and the measurement applications section of Draper and Marcos (1990) each have a series of articles on some of these newer statistical approaches, such as covariance structural modeling (especially linear structural relationships), panel analysis, logistic regression, cluster analysis, log-linear techniques for sequential analysis, and various causal modeling techniques. Each article is written for child or family researchers (rather than other statisticians!)—that is, researchers who

understand well the complexity of problems that have not been adequately captured by traditional statistical methods, but who are unfa-
miliar with some of the assumptions and rationales underlying each new
technique. They are very valuable issues and should be consulted by
those who wish to know more about these new techniques. Continued
flexibility in the use, interpretation, and creation of data analysis approaches will be important in helping family researchers capture the
notions inherent in their theories.

EXERCISES

1. Given the following brief data set, in which each family member received
   a score (possible range, 0-20) on some family construct, compute/note for
   each family: the mean score, the most extreme scores (both high and low),
   and a difference score between mothers and fathers and between the two
   children. Discuss the differences in these methods in terms of how they
   describe the families. First, rank the families high to low based on each
   kind of score. Do the families appear in similar ranks using the four
   different scores? Next, "eyeball" your data and decide which families look
   similar on the basis of each computed measure. Do any of the four scores
   derived match your "eyeball" assessment? In short, if each type of measure
   were basically the same, each measure should result in the families being
   ranked in the same order. Did this happen? If not, why not? Does one type
   of measure show a lot more or less variance than others? Now go back and
   try to think of a construct that might best be measured by each of these
   summary scores (i.e., mean, extreme high, extreme low, mother-father
   difference, child 1-child 2 difference).

Family	Mother	Father	Child 1	Child 2
1	10	7	5	11
2	19	18	15	4
3	15	14	9	13
4	4	5	2	6
5	7	8	7	8
6	16	15	17	14
7	9	12	2	20
8	6	7	20	1

2. Think of a family research question of interest to you. Define an outcome
   variable (or set of variables) and draw a diagram of *all* the influences you
   think are likely to affect this outcome variable. Also include influences that
   probably affect the influences even if the direct effect on the outcome may
   be small. Use your own judgment and what you have learned from various

psychological theories to fill in the diagram completely. Indicate by arrows the direction/directions of effect you think are likely. Once you have a complex diagram, how could you go about assessing the relationships among the variables? How many sources would be needed to get an accurate appraisal of each construct? Is one source better than the other possible ones? Are hypothesized effects all unidirectional in your model? Can you empirically test this unidirectionality? Are the hypothesized effects all linear? Can you test this? Are there relationships in your model which you do not know how to capture statistically? What you have just done is the preliminary work on a causal model.

RECOMMENDED READING

Bakeman, R., & Gottman, J. M. (1986). *Observing interaction: An introduction to sequential analysis.* Cambridge: Cambridge University Press.

Draper, T. W., & Marcos, A. C. (1990). *Family variables: Conceptualization, measurement, and use.* Newbury Park, CA: Sage.

Fisher, L., Kokes, R. F., Ransom, D. C., Phillips, S. L., & Rudd, P. (1985). Alternative strategies for creating "relational" family data. *Family Process, 24,* 213-224.

7

Challenges for Family Researchers

Starting with the traditional methods of those who study individuals, modifying them, first slightly and then more and more radically, family researchers have begun to use new tools to build a literature that addresses the questions raised by their theories. We are in the middle of an evolving process of methodological development, where much progress has been made, but many challenges remain. Because family study is a complex endeavor, approachable from many points of view, this development will necessarily be multifaceted and at times divergent in direction. This pluralism and diversity is good, we believe, even if it temporarily diffuses the strength of family research contributions, for it adds to a solid foundation for understanding family process. We list below some general suggestions for future development.

1. While the notion of a single, unifying theory of family development is attractive in some respects, it is both unlikely to appear in the near future and, we think, is not critical to the field. What is important is that family researchers work within some specified or evolving theoretical framework, and that similarities among theories be recognized where they exist. Streamlining and integrating theories should be considered, but not at the cost of oversimplification. Parsimony should be balanced with maintenance of richness in our endeavor to describe complex family process as clearly as possible.

2. The great contribution of family researchers has been their ability to study more than one person in a family at a time, although most have still been quite restrained in the number of family members they have studied. This has been an entirely appropriate choice, given the methods available; every time an extra person is added to a conversation that will be coded into categories, for example, the system gets much more complex. More self-report accounts of a family complicate the task of using the family as a unit of analysis; even going from the study of dyads to triads was a major advance. Still, continued progress must be made in developing ways to include all relevant family members, as theories demand. This may require the development of more sophisticated technical equipment, more intricate statistical procedures, and/or the choice of more global coding or rating.

In addition, qualitative approaches have the potential to supplement and reorient our current understanding of family complexity.

3. Similarly, we urge that attention be paid to developing methods of studying and understanding less traditional family forms. This will involve acknowledging their importance, proposing ideas about how they work, establishing sampling guidelines and selection criteria, and developing methods that will tap the relevant constructs.

4. Although each approach to the study of the family includes constructs specific to it, there are some constructs that, in some form or other, are widely used. Enmeshment, marital stability, and parental warmth, for example, are aspects of family dynamics that are often discussed in family models, but for which there is no standard measure. Developing a commonly acknowledged standard of assessment (that may consist of several measures) for each of these constructs would facilitate cross-study comparison and thus add immeasurably to the building of empirical models.

5. The step from proposing the importance of a particular construct to demonstrating how to measure it has been shown to be impressively large. While this is, perhaps, no more true for family research than other types of research, it is unusually pressing for family researchers because of the diversity of new models presently being pursued, each of which includes a large number of underdeveloped constructs. We advocate the continued use of multiple measurement, but then suggest that more direct attention be paid to ways to combine information from various sources and how to understand disagreement across measures or informants.

6. Quantitative researchers will probably increasingly rely on complex statistical procedures to describe full models of family process. The gap between the kinds/amount of data family researchers currently gather and the demands of available statistics must be narrowed, from one end or the other, or both. Simultaneously, the potential of qualitative research methods to circumvent these problems, to address complexity in a completely new way, should be explored.

CONCLUSION

We believe these are some of the areas of exciting new development in the field of family research. Others will surely evolve from solutions and attempted solutions to these problems. The historical factors that led to the current complexion of family research (e.g., the development of videotape methodology, the increased sophistication and accessibility of computers and statistical models, the challenges posed by new forms of families, the increased value on ecological validity, the new clinical and theoretical frameworks) will be followed by other important developments, with unforeseen implications for family research. Thus, like families, family study will continue its path through development, changing with maturity and reflecting sociocultural context. It may take on new "members" (new theories, new methods) and lose old ones, with all the difficult reorganization that accompanies such changes. If it is healthy, as we believe it now is, it will effect these changes with flexibility and profit.

References

Achenbach, T. (1982). Research methods in developmental psychopathology. In P. C. Kendall & J. N. Butcher (Eds.), *Handbook of research methods in clinical psychology* (pp. 569-589). New York: John Wiley.

Achenbach, T. M., McConaughy, S. H., & Howell, C. T. (1987). Child/adolescent behavioral and emotional problems: Implications of cross-informant correlations for situational specificity. *Psychological Bulletin, 101,* 213-232.

Allport, G. W. (Ed.). (1965). *Letters from Jenny.* New York: Harcourt, Brace, & World.

Anastasi, A. (1988). *Psychological testing* (6th ed.). New York: Macmillan.

Bakeman, R., & Gottman, J. M. (1986). *Observing interaction: An introduction to sequential analysis.* Cambridge: Cambridge University Press.

Bales, R. F. (1950). *Interaction process analysis.* Reading, MA: Addison-Wesley.

Bar-Yam Hassan, A. (1989, March). Beyond Erikson: Stages of interpersonal development and their manifestations in young adulthood. In K. M. White (Chair), *Individuals in close relationships: Empirical and conceptual approaches.* Symposium presented at the Annual Meeting of the Eastern Psychological Association, Boston.

Baum, C. G., Forehand, R., & Zegiob, L. E. (1979). A review of observer reactivity in adult-child interactions. *Journal of Behavioral Assessment, 1,* 167-178.

Beavers, W. R. (1976). A theoretical basis for family evaluation. In J. M. Lewis, W. R. Beavers, J. T. Gossett, & V. A. Phillips (Eds.), *No single thread: Psychological health in family systems* (pp. 46-82). New York: Brunner/Mazel.

Beavers, W. R. (1977). *Psychotherapy and growth: A family systems perspective.* New York: Brunner/Mazel.

Beavers, W. R. (1982). Healthy, midrange, and severely dysfunctional families. In F. Walsh (Ed.), *Normal family processes* (pp. 45-66). New York: Guilford.

Beavers, W. R., & Voeller, M. N. (1983). Family models: Comparing and contrasting the Olson circumplex model with the Beavers systems model. *Family Process, 22,* 85-98.

Bell, D. C., & Bell, L. G. (1989). Micro and macro measurement of family systems concepts. *Journal of Family Psychology, 3,* 137-157.

Bell, D. C., Bell, L. G., & Cornwell, C. (1982). *Interaction process coding scheme.* Unpublished manuscript. Houston: University of Houston at Clear Lake City.

Bell, G., Cornwell, C., & Bell, D. C. (1983). *Global Scales.* Houston: University of Houston-Clearlake. (ERIC No. ED248420).

Bell, R. Q. (1982). *Parent/adolescent relationships in families with runaways: Interaction types and the circumplex model.* Unpublished doctoral dissertation, University of Minnesota.

Bennett, L. A., Wolin, S. J., Reiss, D., & Teitelbaum, M. P. H. (1987). Couples at risk for transmission of alcoholism: Protective influences. *Family Process, 26,* 111-129.

Bernard, J. (1982). *The future of marriage.* New Haven, CT: Yale University.

Biddle, B. J., & Marlin, M. M. (1987). Causality, confirmation, credulity, and structural equation modeling. *Child Development, 58,* 4-17.

Birchler, G. R., Weiss, R. L., & Vincent, J. P. (1975). Multimethod analysis of social reinforcement exchange between maritally distressed and nondistressed spouse and stranger dyads. *Journal of Personality and Social Psychology, 31,* 349-360.

Blinn, L. (1988). The Family Photo Assessment Process (FPAP): A method for validating cross-cultural comparisons of family social identities. *Journal of Comparative Family Studies, 19*(1), 17-35.

Block, J. H. (1966). *The Child-Rearing Practices Report (CRPR): A set of Q items for the description of parental socialization attitudes and values.* Unpublished scoring manual, University of California, Berkeley.

Block, J. H. (1973). Conceptions of sex role: Some cross cultural and longitudinal perspectives. *American Psychologist, 28,* 512-526.

Bryant, A. L., & Coleman, M. (1988). The black family as portrayed in introductory marriage and family textbooks. *Family Relations, 37,* 255-259.

Burr, W. R., Hill, R., Nye, F. I., & Reiss, I. L. (Eds.). (1979a). *Contemporary theories about the family* (Vol. 1). New York: Free Press.

Burr, W. R., Hill, R., Nye, F. I., & Reiss, I. L. (Eds.). (1979b). *Contemporary theories about the family* (Vol. 2). New York: Free Press.

Carlson, C. I., & Grotevant, H. D. (1987a). A comparative review of family rating scales: Guidelines for clinicians and researchers. *Journal of Family Psychology, 1*(1), 23-47.

Carlson, C. I., & Grotevant, H. D. (1987b). Rejoinder: The challenges of reconciling family theory with method. *Journal of Family Psychology, 1*(1), 62-65.

Carmines, E. G., & Zeller, R. A. (1979). Reliability and validity assessment. *Quantitative applications in the social sciences* (No. 17). Beverly Hills, CA: Sage.

Chamberlain, P., & Bank, L. (1989). Commentary: Toward an integration of macro and micro measurement systems for the researcher and clinician. *Journal of Family Psychology, 3,* 199-205.

Christensen, A., & Arrington, A. (1987). Research issues and strategies. In T. Jacob (Ed.), *Family interaction and psychopathology: Theories, methods, and findings* (pp. 259-296). New York: Plenum.

Colby, A. (1982). The use of secondary analysis in the study of women and social change. *Journal of Social Issues, 38*(1), 119-123.

Condon, S. L., Cooper, C. R., & Grotevant, H. D. (1984). Manual for the analysis of family discourse. *Psychological Documents, 14*(8; MS No. 2616).

Copeland, A. P. (1990). *Family alliances and children's behavioral style.* Study in progress.

Copeland, A. P., Stewart, A. J., & Healy, J. M. (1989, January). *Parentified children's experience following divorce.* Paper presented at the Society for Research in Child and Adolescent Psychopathology, Miami.

Costos, D. (1986). Sex role identity in young adults: Its parental antecedents and relation to ego development. *Journal of Personality and Social Psychology, 50,* 602-611.

Cousins, P. C., & Power, T. G. (1986). Quantifying family process: Issues in the analysis of interaction sequences. *Family Process, 25,* 89-105.

Cowan, P. A. (1987). The need for theoretical and methodological integrations in family research. *Journal of Family Psychology, 1*(1), 48-50.

Coyne, J. C. (1987). Some issues in the assessment of family patterns. *Journal of Family Psychology, 1*(1), 51-57.

Cromwell, R. E., & Peterson, G. W. (1983). Multisystem-multimethod family assessment in clinical contexts. *Family Process, 22,* 147-163.

Doane, J. A. (1978). Family interaction and communication deviance in disturbed and normal families. *Family Process, 17*, 357-373.

Doane, J. A., Goldstein, M. J., & Rodenick, E. H. (1981). Parental patterns of affective style and the development of schizophrenia spectrum disorders. *Family Process, 20*, 337-349.

Draper, T. W., & Marcos, A. C. (1990). *Family variables: Conceptualization, measurement, and use.* Newbury Park, CA: Sage.

Elder, G. J., Jr. (1974). *Children of the Great Depression.* Chicago: University of Chicago Press.

Elder, G. J., Jr., Nguyen, T. V., & Caspi, A. (1985). Linking family hardship to children's lives. *Child Development, 56*, 361-375.

Epstein, N. B., Bishop, D. S., & Levine, S. (1978). The McMaster model of family functioning. *Journal of Marriage and Family Counseling, 4*(4), 19-31.

Erez, E., & Tontodonato, P. (1989). Patterns of reported parent-child abuse and police response. *Journal of Family Violence, 4*, 143-159.

Feldman, S. S., Wentzel, K. R., & Gehring, T. M. (1989). A comparison of the views of mothers, fathers, and pre-adolescents about family cohesion and power. *Journal of Family Psychology, 3*(1), 39-60.

Ferreira, A. J. (1963). Decision-making in normal and pathological families. *Archives of General Psychiatry, 2*, 68-73.

Fetterman, D. (1989) *Ethnography: Step by step.* Newbury Park, CA: Sage.

Filsinger, E. E. (1983). Choices among marital observation coding systems. *Family Process, 22*, 317-335.

Filsinger, E. E. (1990). Empirical typology, cluster analysis, and family-level measurement. In T. W. Draper & A. C. Marcos (Eds.), *Family variables: Conceptualization, measurement, and use* (pp. 90-104). Newbury Park, CA: Sage.

Fisher, L. (1987). Observational rating scales: Supplementary comments. *Journal of Family Psychology, 1*(1), 58-61.

Fisher, L., Kokes, R. F., Ransom, D. C., Phillips, S. L., & Rudd, P. (1985). Alternative strategies for creating "relational" family data. *Family Process, 24*, 213-224.

Fowler, F. J., Jr. (1989). *Survey research methods.* Newbury Park, CA: Sage.

Fowler, P. C. (1982a). Factor structure of the Family Environment Scale: Effects of social desirabilty. *Journal of Clinical Psychology, 38*, 285-292.

Fowler, P. C. (1982b). Relationship of family environment and personality characteristics: Canonical analyses of self-attributions. *Journal of Clinical Psychology, 38*, 804-810.

Gilbert, R., & Christensen, A. (1985). Observational assessment of marital and family interaction: Methodological considerations. In L. L'Abate (Ed.), *The handbook of family psychology and therapy* (Vol. 2, pp. 961-987). Homewood, IL: Dorsey.

Gilbert, R., Saltar, K., Deskin, J., Karagozian, A., Severance, G., & Christensen, A. (1981). *Family Alliances Coding System Manual (FACS).* Unpublished manuscript.

Godwin, D. D. (1988). Causal modeling in family research. *Journal of Marriage and the Family, 50*, 917-927.

Gottman, J. M. (1979). *Marital interaction: Empirical investigations.* New York: Academic Press.

Gottman, J. M., & Krokoff, L. J. (1989). Marital interaction and satisfaction: A longitudinal view. *Journal of Consulting and Clinical Psychology, 57*(1), 47-52.

Gottman, J. M., Markman, H. J., & Notarius, C. I. (1977). The topography of marital conflict: A sequential analysis of verbal and nonverbal behavior. *Journal of Marriage and the Family, 39,* 361-377.

Grotevant, H. D. (1989). The role of theory in guiding family assessment. *Journal of Family Psychology, 3*(2), 104-117.

Grotevant, H. D., & Carlson, C. I. (1987). Family interaction coding systems: A descriptive review. *Family Process, 26,* 49-74.

Grotevant, H. D., & Carlson, C. I. (1988). *Family assessment: A guide to methods and measures.* New York: Guilford.

Grotevant, H. D., & Cooper, C. R. (1985). Patterns of interaction in family relationships and the development of identity exploration. *Child Development, 56,* 415-428.

Hampson, R. B., Beavers, W. R., & Hulgus, Y. F. (1989) Insiders' and outsiders' views of family: The assessment of family competence and style. *Journal of Family Psychology, 3*(2), 118-136.

Hauser, S. T., Powers, S. I., Noam, G. G., Jacobson, A. M., Weiss, B., & Follansbee, D. J. (1984). Familial contexts of adolescent ego development. *Child Development, 55,* 195-213.

Hauser, S. T., Powers, S. I., Weiss, B., Follansbee, D., & Bernstein, E. (1983). *Family constraining and enabling coding system (CECS) manual.* Unpublished manuscript, Boston.

Haynes, S. N., Follingstad, D. R., & Sullivan, J. C. (1979). Assessment of marital satisfaction and interaction. *Journal of Consulting and Clinical Psychology, 47,* 789-791.

Haynes, S. N., & Horn, W. (1982). Reactivity in behavioral observation: A review. *Behavioral Assessment, 4,* 369-385.

Hinde, R. (1979). *Towards understanding relationships.* New York: Academic Press.

Hochschild, A. (1989). *The second shift: Working parents and the revolution at home.* New York: Viking.

Hops, H., Wills, T. A., Patterson, G. R., & Weiss, R. L. (1972). *Marital Interaction Coding System.* Eugene: Oregon Research Institute.

Huston, T. L., & Robins, E. (1982). Conceptual and methodological issues in studying close relationships. *Journal of Marriage and the Family, 44,* 901-925.

Huston, T. L., Robins, E., Atkinson J., & McHale, S. M. (1987). Surveying the landscape of marital behavior: A behavioral self-report approach to studying marriage. In S. Oskamp (Ed.), *Family processes and problems: Social psychological aspects.* Applied Social Psychology Annual, Vol. 7, 45-72.

Jackson, J. S., Tucker, M. B., & Bowman, P. J. (1982). Conceptual and methodological issues in survey research on black Americans. In W. T. Lui (Ed.), *Methodological problems in minority research.* Chicago: Pacific/Asian American Mental Health Center.

Jacob, T. (1975). Family interaction in disturbed and normal families: A methodological and substantive review. *Psychological Bulletin, 82,* 33-65.

Jacob, T. (Ed.). (1987). *Family interaction and psychopathology: Theories, methods, and findings.* New York: Plenum.

Jacobson, N. S. (1977). Problem solving and contingency contracting in the treatment of marital discord. *Journal of Consulting and Clinical Psychology, 45,* 92-100.

Jayaratne, T. E., & Stewart, A. J. (in press). Quantitative and qualitative methods in the social sciences: Current feminist issues and practical strategies. In M. M. Fonow & J. A. Cook (Eds.), *Beyond methodology.* Bloomington: Indiana University Press.

Johnson, D. R., & Booth, A. (1990). Rural economic decline and marital quality: A panel study of farm marriages. *Family Relations, 39,* 159-165.

Johnson, S. M., & Bolstad, O. D. (1975). Reactivity to home observation: A comparison of audiorecorded behavior with observers present or absent. *Journal of Applied Behavior Analysis, 8,* 181-185.

Johnson, S. M., & Lobitz, G. A. (1974). Parental manipulations of child behavior in home observations. *Journal of Applied Behavior Analysis, 7,* 23-31.

Jones, M. C., Bayley, N., Macfarlane, J. W., & Honzik, M. P. (1971). *The course of human development.* Waltham, MA: Xerox College Publishing.

Kabacoff, R. I., Miller, I. W., Bishop, D. S., Epstein, N. B., & Keitner, G. I. (1990). A psychometric study of the McMaster Family Assessment Device in psychiatric, medical and nonclinical samples. *Journal of Family Psychology, 3,* 431-439.

Kazdin, A. E. (1982). Observer effects: Reactivity of direct observation. In D. P. Hartmann (Ed.), *Using observers to study behavior* (pp. 5-19). San Francisco: Jossey-Bass.

Klein, D. M., & Hill, R. (1979). Determinants of family problem-solving effectiveness. In W. R. Burr, R. Hill, F. I. Nye, & I. L. Reiss (Eds.), *Contemporary theories about the family* (Vol. 1; pp. 493-548). New York: Free Press.

Koo, H. P., Suchindran, C. M., & Griffith, J. D. (1987). The completion of childbearing: Change and variation in timing. *Journal of Marriage and the Family, 49,* 281-293.

L'Abate, L. (Ed.). (1985). *The handbook of family psychology and therapy* (Vol. 1, 2). Homewood, IL: Dorsey.

Larsen, A., & Olson, D. H. (1990). Capturing the complexity of family systems: Integrating family theory, family scores, and family analysis. In T. W. Draper & A. C. Marcos (Eds.), *Family variables: Conceptualization, measurement, and use* (pp. 19-47). Newbury Park, CA: Sage.

Layton, L. (1988, May). *Gender differences in narcissism.* Paper presented at the annual meeting of the Massachusetts Psychological Association, Boston.

Lewis, J. M., Beavers, W. R., Gossett, J. T., & Phillips, V. A. (1976). *No single thread.* New York: Brunner/Mazel.

Liker, J., & Elder, G. (1983). Economic hardship and marital relations in the 1930s. *American Sociological Review, 48,* 343-359.

Lobitz, W. C., & Johnson, S. M. (1975). Parental manipulation of the behavior of normal and deviant children. *Child Development, 46,* 719-726.

Locke, H. J., & Wallace, K. M. (1959). Short marital-adjustment and prediction tests: Their reliability and validity. *Marriage and Family Living,* 251-255.

Loevinger, J. (1976). *Ego development: Conceptions and theories.* San Francisco: Jossey-Bass.

Loveland, N. T., Wynne, L. C., & Singer, M. T. (1963). The family Rorschach: A new method for studying family interaction. *Family Process, 2,* 187-215.

Markman, H. J., & Notarius, C. I. (1987). Coding marital and family interaction: Current status. In T. Jacob (Ed.), *Family interaction and psychopathology: Theories, methods, and findings* (pp. 329-390). New York: Plenum.

Martin, B. (1987). Developmental perspectives on family theory and psychopathology. In T. Jacob (Ed.), *Family interaction and psychopathology* (pp. 163-202). New York: Plenum.

Martin, J. A. (1987). Structural equation modeling: A guide for the perplexed. *Child Development, 58*(1), 33-37.

Mash, E. J., & Barkley, R. A. (1986). Assessment of family interaction with the Response-Class Matrix. In R. J. Prinz (Ed.), *Advances in behavioral assessment of children and families* (Vol. 2, pp. 29-67). Greenwich, CT: JAI.

Mash, E. J., Terdal, L. G., & Anderson, K. (1973). The Response-Class Matrix: A procedure for recording parent-child interactions. *Journal of Consulting and Clinical Psychology, 40,* 163-164.

Massie, H. N. (1978). The early natural history of childhood psychosis: Ten cases studied by analysis of family home movies of the infancies of the children. *Journal of the American Academy of Child Psychiatry, 17,* 29-45.

Massie, H. N. (1980). Pathological interactions in infancy. In T. M. Field, S. Goldberg, D. Stern, & A. M. Sostek (Eds.), *High-risk infants and children: Adult and peer interactions* (pp. 79-97). New York: Academic Press.

Milner, J. S. (1986). *The Child Abuse Potential Inventory: Manual* (2nd ed.). Webster, NC: Psytec Corporation.

Milner, J. S. & Wimberley, R. C. (1979). An inventory for the identification of child abusers. *Journal of Clinical Psychology, 35,* 95-100.

Mishler, E. G., & Waxler, N. W. (1968). *Interaction in families: An experimental study of family processes and schizophrenia.* New York: John Wiley.

Monahan, M. (1989, March). Empathy and its corrrelates in young adults. In K. M. White (Chair), *Individuals in close relationships: Empirical and conceptual approaches.* Symposium presented at the Annual Meeting of the Eastern Psychological Association, Boston.

Moos, R. H. (1974). *Combined preliminary manual for the family, work and group environment scales.* Palo Alto, CA: Consulting Psychologists Press.

Moos, R. H., & Moos B. (1981). *Family Environment Scale manual.* Palo Alto, CA: Consulting Psychologists Press.

Moos, R. H., & Spinrad, S. (1984). *The Social Climate Scales: An annotated bibliography.* Palo Alto, CA: Consulting Psychologists Press.

Noller, P., & Shum, D. (1990). The couple version of FACES III: Validity and reliability. *Journal of Family Psychology, 3,* 440-451.

Oliveri, M. E., & Reiss, D. (1984). Family concepts and their measurement: Things are seldom what they seem. *Family Process, 23,* 33-48.

Olson, D. H. (1977). Insiders' and outsiders' views of relationships: Research and strategies. In G. Levinger & H. Raush (Eds.), *Close relationships* (pp. 115-136). Amherst: University of Massachusetts Press.

Olson, D. H. (1985). Commentary: Struggling with congruence across theoretical models and methods. *Family Process, 24,* 203-207.

Olson, D. H. (1990). Reply to Noller and Shum. *Journal of Family Psychology, 3,* 452-453.

Olson, D. H., Portner, J., & Lavee, Y. (1985). *FACES III.* St. Paul: Family Social Science, University of Minnesota.

Olson, D. H., Russell, C. S., & Sprenkle, D. H. (1979). Circumplex model of marital and family systems: 2. Empirical studies and clinical intervention. In J. Vincent (Ed.), *Advances in family interaction, assessment and theory.* Greenwich, CT: JAI.

Olson, D. H., Russell, C. S., & Sprenkle, D. H. (1983). Circumplex model of marital and family systems: 4. Theoretical update. *Family Process, 22,* 69-83.

Olson, D. H., Sprenkle, D. H., & Russell, C. S. (1979). Circumplex model of marital and family systems: 1. Cohesion and adaptability dimensions, family types, and clinical applications. *Family Process, 18,* 3-28.

Oster, S. M. (1987). A note on the determinants of alimony. *Journal of Marriage and the Family, 49,* 81-86.

Ozer, D. J. (1989). Construct validity in personality assessment. In D. Buss & N. Cantor (Eds.), *Personality psychology: Recent trends and emerging directions* (pp. 224-234). New York: Springer-Verlag.

Patterson, G. R. (1982). *Coerceive family process.* Eugene, OR: Castilia.

Patterson, G. R. (1984). Microsocial process: A view from the boundary. In J. C. Masters & K. Yarkin-Levin (Eds.), *Boundary areas in social and developmental psychology* (pp. 24-35). New York: Academic Press.

Patterson, G. R., Ray, R. S., Shaw, D. A., & Cobb, J. A. (1969). *Manual for coding of family interactions* (rev. ed.). New York: Microfiche Publications.

Paul, E. (1989, August). *Intimacy development in young adulthood: A differential approach to relationship experiences.* Paper presented at the annual meeting of the American Psychological Association, New Orleans.

Pedhazur, E. J. (1982). *Multiple regression in behavioral research: Explanation and prediction* (2nd ed.). New York: Holt, Rinehart & Winston.

Peterson, D. R. (1979). Assessing interpersonal relationships by means of interaction records. *Behavioral Assessment, 1,* 221-236.

Pogue-Geile, M. F., & Rose, R. J. (1987). Psychopathology: A behavior genetic perspective. In T. Jacob (Ed.), *Family interaction and psychopathology* (pp. 629-650). New York: Plenum.

Portner, J. (1981). *Parent/adolescent relationships: Interaction types and the circumplex model.* Unpublished doctoral dissertation, Family Social Science, University of Minnesota.

Rank, M. R. (1987). The formation and dissolution of marriages in the welfare population. *Journal of Marriage and the Family, 49,* 15-20.

Ransom, D. C., Fisher, L., Phillips, S., Kokes, R. F., & Weiss, R. (1990). The logic of measurement in family research. In T. W. Draper & A. C. Marcos (Eds.), *Family variables: Conceptualization, measurement, and use* (pp. 48-63). Newbury Park, CA: Sage.

Reid, J. B. (Ed.). (1978). *A social learning approach to family intervention. Vol. 2: Observation in home settings.* Eugene, OR: Castalia.

Reid, J. B., Baldwin, D. V., Patterson, G. R., & Dishion, T. J. (1988). Observations in the assessment of childhood disorders. In M. Rutter, A. H. Tuma, & I. S. Lann (Eds.), *Assessment and diagnosis in child psychopathology* (pp. 156-195). London: Fulton.

Reinharz, S. (1984). *On becoming a social scientist: From survey research and participant observation to experiential analysis.* New Brunswick, NJ: Transaction Books.

Reiss, D. (1981). *The family's construction of reality.* Cambridge, MA: Harvard University Press.

Riskin, J. (1982). Research on "nonlabeled" families: A longitudinal study. In F. Walsh (Ed.), *Normal family process* (pp. 67-93). New York: Guilford.

Riskin, J., & Faunce, E. E. (1972). An evaluative review of family interaction research. *Family Process, 11,* 365-456.

Roberts, G. C., Block, J. H., & Block, J. (1984). Continuity and change in parents' child-rearing practices. *Child Development, 55,* 586-597.

Robinson, E. A., & Eyberg, S. M. (1981). The dyadic parent-child interaction coding system: Standardization and validation. *Journal of Consulting and Clinical Psychology, 49,* 245-250.

Robinson, E. A., & Jacobson, N. S. (1987). Social learning theory and family psychopathology: A Kantian model in behaviorism? In T. Jacob (Ed.), *Family interaction and psychopathology* (pp. 117-162). New York: Plenum.

Rogers, L. E., Millar, F. E., & Bavelas, J. B. (1985). Methods for analyzing marital conflict discourse: Implications of a systems approach. *Family Process, 24,* 175-187.

Schumm, W., Barnes, H. L., Bollman, S. R., Jurich, A. P., & Milliken, G. A. (1984, October). *Approaches to the statistical analysis of family data.* Paper presented at meeting of National Council on Family Relations, San Francisco.

Sears, R. R. (1979, June). Mark Twain's separation anxiety. *Psychology Today,* pp. 100-104.

Siegel, S. (1956). *Nonparametric statistics for the behavioral sciences.* New York: McGraw-Hill.

Sigafoos, A., & Reiss, D. (1985). Rejoinder: Counterperspectives on family measurement: Clarifying the pragmatic interpretation of research methods. *Family Process, 24,* 207-211.

Sigafoos, A., Reiss, D., Rich, J., & Douglas, E. (1985). Pragmatics in the measurement of family functioning: An interpretive framework for methodology. *Family Process, 24,* 189-203.

Singer, M., & Wynne, L. (1966). Principles for scoring communication defects and deviances in parents of schizophrenics: Rorschach and TAT scoring manuals. *Psychiatry, 29,* 260-288.

Skinner, H. A., Steinhauer, P. D., & Santa-Barbara, J. (1983). The Family Assessment Measure. *Canadian Journal of Community Mental Health, 2,* 91-105.

Sklover, S., White, K. M., & Wenar, C. (1988). *Perceived child-rearing practices, intimacy maturity, and the maturity of young adults' relationships with their parents.* Unpublished manuscript.

Spanier, G. B. (1973). Whose marital adjustment?: A research note. *Sociological Inquiry, 43,* 95-96.

Spanier, G. B. (1976). Measuring dyadic adjustment: New scales for assessing the quality of marriage and similar dyads. *Journal of Marriage and the Family, 38,* 15-28.

Spanier, G. B., & Cole, C. L. (1976). Toward clarification of marital adjustment. *International Journal of the Sociology of the Family, 6,* 121-146.

Sprey, J. (1988). Current theorizing on the family: An appraisal. *Journal of Marriage and the Family, 50,* 875-890.

Steinglass, P. (1976). *Home Observation Assessment Method.* Unpublished manuscript, Center for Family Research, Washington, DC.

Steinglass, P. (1979). The home observation assessment method (HOAM): Real-time observations of families in their homes. *Family Process, 18,* 337-354.

Steinglass, P. (1987). A systems view of family interaction and psychopathology. In T. Jacob (Ed.), *Family interaction and psychopathology* (pp. 25-65). New York: Plenum.

Steinglass, P., Tislenko, L., & Reiss, D. (1985). Stability/instability in the alcoholic marriage: The interrelationships between course of alcoholism, family process, and marital outcome. *Family Process, 24,* 365-376.

Steirlin, H. (1974). *Separating parents and adolescents.* New York: Quadrangle.

Stewart, A. J., Franz, C., & Layton, L. (1988). The changing self: Using personal documents to study lives. *Journal of Personality, 56*(1), 41-74.

Stewart, D. W. (1984). *Secondary research: Information sources and methods.* Beverly Hills, CA: Sage.

Straus, M. A. (1979). Measuring intrafamily conflict and violence: The Conflict Tactics (CT) Scales. *Journal of Marriage and the Family, 41,* 75-88.

Straus, M. A., & Tallman, I. (1971). SIMFAM: A technique for observational measurement and experimental study of families. In J. Aldous (Ed.), *Family problem solving* (pp. 380-438). Hinsdale, IL: Dryden.

Szinovacz, M. E. (1983). Using couple data as a methodological tool: The case of marital violence. *Journal of Marriage and the Family, 45,* 633-644.

Thomas, D. L., & Wilcox, J. E. (1987). The rise of family theory: A historical and critical analysis. In M. B. Sussman & S. K. Steinmetz (Eds.), *Handbook of marriage and the family* (pp. 81-102). New York: Plenum.

Touliatos, J., Perlmutter, B. F., & Straus, M. A. (Eds.). (1989). *Family measurement techniques.* Newbury Park, CA: Sage.

von Bertalanffy, L. (1968). *General systems theory.* New York: George Braziller.

Vuchinich, S., Emery, R. E., & Cassidy, J. (1988). Family members as third parties in dyadic famiy conflict: Strategies, alliances, and outcomes. *Child Development, 59,* 1293-1302.

Walters, L. H., Pittman, J. F., & Norrel, J. E. (1984). Development of a quantitative measure of a family from self-reports of family members. *Journal of Family Issues.*

Waring, E. M., & Chelune, G. J. (1983). Marital intimacy and self-disclosure. *Journal of Clinical Psychology, 39,* 183-190.

Waring, E. M., McElrath, D., Mitchell, P., & Derry, M. E. (1981). Intimacy and emotional illness in the general population. *Canadian Journal of Psychiatry, 26,* 167-172.

Waring, E. M., & Reddon, J. R. (1983). The measurement of intimacy in marriage: The Waring Intimacy Questionnaire. *Journal of Clinical Psychology, 39,* 53-57.

Webb, E. J., Campbell, D. T., Schwartz, R. D., & Sechrest, L. (1966). *Nonreactive research in the social sciences.* Boston: Houghton Mifflin.

Wechsler, D. (1974). Wechsler Intelligence Scale for Children—Revised. New York: The Psychological Corporation.

Weinrott, M. R., Garrett, B., & Todd, N. (1978). The influence of observer presence on classroom behavior. *Behavior Therapy, 9,* 900-911.

Weiss, R. L., & Summers, K. (1983). The Marital Interaction Coding System: III. In E. E. Filsinger (Ed.), *Marriage and family assessment: A sourcebook for family therapy.* Beverly Hills, CA: Sage.

White, K. M., Houlihan, J., Speisman, J. C., & Costos, D. (1990). Adult development in individuals and relationships. *Journal of Research in Personality, 24,* 371-386.

White, K. M., Speisman, J. C., Costos, D., Jackson, D., & Bartis, S. (in press). *Intimacy scoring manual.* San Rafael, CA: Select Press.

White, K. M., Speisman, J. C., Costos, D., & Smith, A. (1987). Relationship maturity: A conceptual and empirical approach. In J. Meacham (Ed.), *Interpersonal relations: Family, peers, friends. Vol. 18: Contributions to human development.* Basel, Switzerland: Karger.

White, K. M., Speisman, J. C., Jackson, D., Bartis, S., & Costos, D. (1986). Intimacy maturity and its correlates in young married couples. *Journal of Personality and Social Psychology, 50*(1), 152-162.

Wrightsman, L. S. (1981). Personal documents as data in conceptualizing adult personality development. *Personality and Social Psychology Bulletin, 7,* 367-385.

Index

114

About the Authors

Anne P. Copeland received her Ph.D. in clinical psychology in 1977 from the American University in Washington, DC. She is currently Associate Professor of psychology at Boston University, where she teaches courses in child development and child and family clinical psychology. Co-investigator on a longitudinal project of family transformation following parental divorce, she has been able to use this data set to operationalize some important dimensions of family interaction (including parentification, triangulation, spousal conflict, and parental warmth), and to test some aspects of systemic theory that have traditionally been difficult to assess. She is interested in the family and temperament factors that underlie symptoms in children. She has been principal investigator and director of the Boston University family research training program and head of the programs in human development, a doctoral program that integrates the study of personality, social, and developmental psychology.

Kathleen M. White received a B.A. in history from Swarthmore College and an Ed.D. in special education from Boston University. Currently a professor in the Boston University Psychology Department, she is the principal author of several books, including *Adolescence, Research Approaches to Personality,* and *Treating Child Abuse and Family Violence in Hospitals.* A recipient of two grants from the National Institute of Mental Health for her research on family relationships, she has been project director and codirector of an NIMH training grant for training graduate students in family research methods. Her research has focused primarily on maturity in relationships, and she has published many articles on this and related topics. She teaches both graduate and undergraduate courses in family psychology and research methods, and was one of the representative psychologists featured in the American Psychological Association's publication on *Careers in Psychology.*

NOTES

NOTES